Aromatherapy
Treatments

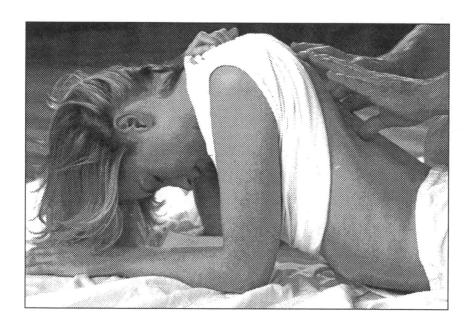

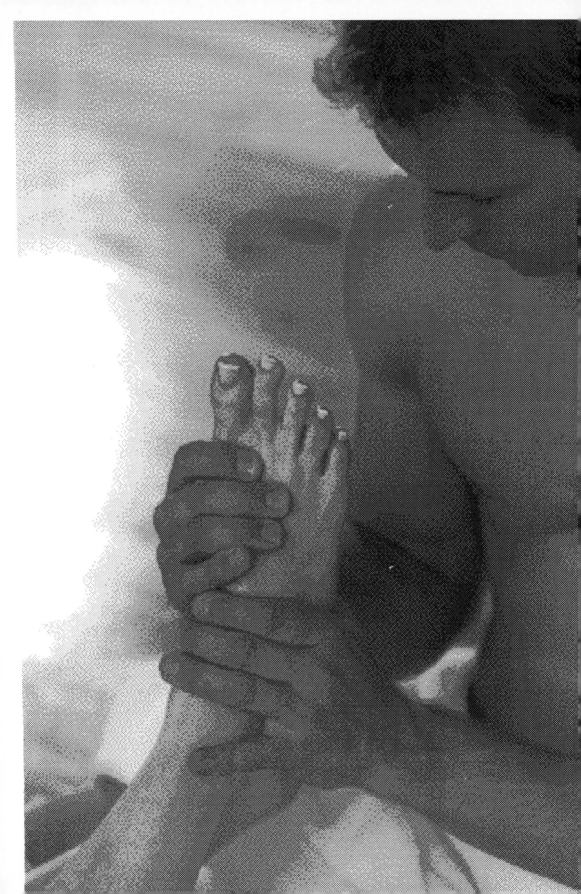

Astrolog ◆ The Quality of Life Series

Aromatherapy Treatments

Marion Wayman

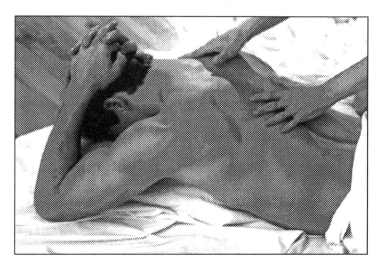

Astrolog Publishing House Ltd.

Cover design: Na'ama Yaffe

All rights reserved to Astrolog Publishing House Ltd.
P.O. Box 1123, Hod Hasharon 45111, Israel
Tel: 972-9-7412044
Fax: 972-9-7442714

© Astrolog Publishing House Ltd. 2004

ISBN 965-494-137-6

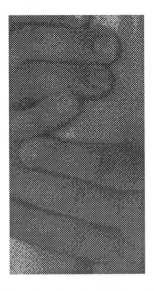

Published by Astrolog Publishing House 2004

Contents

Usual disclaimer

Aromatherapy is a growing field in alternative medicine, beauty care, development of awareness, and other New Age areas. Nowadays, everyone is familiar with the aromatherapy oils, and many people use them in one way or another.

This book aims to broaden the horizon of both professional readers, who use aromatherapy oils on a regular basis, and of readers who are interested in becoming acquainted with the benefit they can derive from these oils.

There are many books that give a detailed list of the aromatherapy oils, as well as the properties (partially therapeutic) that are attributed to these oils. This "inventory" is not repeated here. However, every oil we use is described at length in the chapters on the aromatherapy treatments.

The pictures show the part of the body on which the particular massage technique is performed. They also sometimes illustrate the recommended technique itself.
When massage is not optimal in the aromatherapy treatment, there are no illustrative pictures.
The pictures should be treated as illustration only, and therefore the chapter should be read in its entirety.

1

Introduction

The history of essential oils

From time immemorial, man has searched for ways to utilize the innumerable types of plants found in nature for his benefit – for eating, for healing, and for improving his health, his appearance, and his overall feeling.

Three thousand years BC, the Egyptians had already discovered essential oils. Various methods of treatment using medicinal plants had existed a long time before that, but from that period onward there is evidence of the use of aromatic essences. Many who research the Egyptian mummification methods believe that among the secret ingredients of the mummification substances were various essential oils, one of which could be the cedarwood oil that is familiar to us today. The wealthy women of Egypt also utilized the properties of the essential oils in their beauty creams, perfumes, and skin rejuvenation treatments as part of their legendary beauty care. The Bible, too, mentions frankincense and myrrh, both for ceremonial use as incense and for cosmetic and medicinal use (they were also two of the three gifts presented to the Baby Jesus). Researchers and archeologists believe that the highly-developed trade in essential oils began as early as 4,000 years ago, and they have even found evidence of this in an ancient Babylonian pottery fragment that is about 3,800 years old, and which served as an order form for the import of oils.

Like the Egyptians, both the Greeks and the Romans used essential oils for perfume, healing, and body care, attributing a broad range of properties to the oils – medicinal, cosmetic, and even mystical and religious. To this day, for instance, frankincense oil, which was used in the preparation of incense in the Temple in Jerusalem, is considered to be a superb oil for use during meditation because of its properties, which enhance spiritual openness.

In ancient times, the Egyptians, Greeks, and Romans wrote books about the use of the oils, but only a tiny portion of these writings have survived. Other ancient civilizations were familiar with the properties of the oils, among them Crete, India, and China. It is possible that the Chinese knew about the use of essential oils even before the Egyptians. In Africa, too, massage with essential oils was very common.

There is evidence of the use of essential oils in Europe in the 14th and 15th centuries, even though production methods were different. In Europe, infused oils were used – that is, the petals and other parts of the plant were soaked in hot carrier oil and then drained a few days later, so that a blend of essential oil and carrier oil was obtained. Over time, the use of oils became more common and widespread in Europe, and they were used mainly externally, but sometimes also internally for treating certain internal ailments. In the 17th century, treatment with medicinal plants became very widespread and popular, and was one of the most preferred methods of treatment.

At the same time, and also in the 18th century, many books were written about treatment with plants and essential oils, including recipes and various blends for treating specific diseases and problems. At the beginning of the 19th century, the oils began to be examined scientifically. During this time, books were published describing the multiple properties of the essential oils, some of them checked and tried, for treating various problems. Although at that time, the production of chemical medications had begun, pushing aside the traditional use of medicinal plants, the research into and use of essential oils continued to gain momentum. The essential oil industry also flourished, and many plots of land were allocated for growing the plants that were used in the production of the essential oils.

As for perfumes, there is no doubt that the essential oils have always starred in the composition of the costly substances. Oils such as sandalwood, patchouli, ylang-ylang, jasmine, and, of course, rose, are just a few of the oils that have long been used in the perfume industry because of their marvelous fragrance. The use of cedarwood oil is widespread in fragrances for men.

Part of the renown enjoyed by essential oils today, thanks to their effective therapeutic and healing abilities, can be credited to Réné Gattefossé, who examined and investigated the antiseptic properties of the essential oils. Réné-Maurice Gattefossé was a French cosmetic chemist who experimented with the inclusion of antiseptic properties in cosmetics, and discovered that some of the essential oils possessed antiseptic powers that were greater than those of various chemical substances. Gattefossé experienced the marvelous healing capacity of the oils firsthand when, during one of his chemical experiments, there was an explosion in his laboratory, and as a result one of his hands was burned. Gattefossé immediately immersed his hand in a vat of pure lavender oil – the oil whose properties he had been investigating at the time – and to his amazement, the burn healed rapidly, leaving no marks, scars, or infection. It was Gattefossé who coined the phrase "aromatic therapy" in the title of his first book, which was published in 1928. The book evoked a great deal of interest among scientists and researchers, and it did not take long for many other books, studies, and articles on essential oils, their properties, and their uses, to appear.

As a self-standing treatment, aromatic therapy started off as a treatment for wounds sustained during World War II, when a French physician – Dr. Jean Valnet – treated battlefield wounds and discovered the amazing properties of essential oils.

The first "civilian" clinic for treatment with essential oils was opened by Marguerite Maury, a biochemist who was interested in the oils for cosmetic treatments. Although the external use of essential oils has been known for thousands of years, it was Marguerite Maury who made them as popular, well-known, and widespread, as they are today, when she performed in-depth studies of the action, properties, and effect of the oils. She set up a clinic for treatment with essential oils in England, where she developed the method of massage with essential oils, and was one of the first to combine this massage with medical cosmetic treatment and with treatments for skin problems.

Since then, many researchers, practitioners, and healers have been using essential oils, developing and investigating their methods of use, and to this day continue developing new techniques and treatment methods using essential oils, whose marvelous therapeutic properties affect body, mind, and spirit.

The holistic principle behind treating with essential oils

One of the most important principles in aromatherapy is the holistic principle. In other words, the practitioner (or a person who administers self-treatment) must focus on a client's whole body – all of his problems or states of physical or mental imbalance. The treatment does not relate only to physical or emotional or mental symptoms, but always seeks to be a full body-mind treatment. Indeed, if we look at the oils themselves, we can see that most of them can treat a number of systems, and possess varied and diverse properties. A large number of the oils that are used for treating physical problems also have a significant effect on the emotional level. It must be remembered that both on the emotional and on the physical levels, it is always important to find the reason for or cause of the problem.

The symptoms of various problems can be treated very effectively with essential oils, which provide substantial relief. However, if the practitioner (or the person himself) examines the reason for or the cause of the problem, and can find the link between body and mind and to the interaction between them, he will be able to devise a more effective treatment that concentrates on the causes and not on the external symptoms. He may be able to treat the root of the problem and reach an overall solution rather than simply relieve the symptoms. When aromatherapy is combined with nutrition, treatment of the emotional layers using various techniques (guided imagery, positive thinking, healing, psychotherapy, Bach flower remedies, etc.), and of the physical layers using additional techniques (massage, reflexology, Shiatsu, and so on), and sometimes, in the case of certain diseases, administered in parallel to conventional medical care (preferably in conjunction with the physician involved), the results can be surprisingly successful.

Regarding the holistic principle, it is a good idea to compile a comprehensive list of the client's complaints – even if he has come because of a single or specific complaint – and find the oils that will treat all or most of them.

For instance, when a client comes to us suffering from back pain, which is the main symptom bothering him, we look for the oils that treat this problem. At the same time, we pay attention to the client's other complaints – for example, difficulty in falling asleep at night, menstrual pains, nervousness, and hypersensitivity. When we prepare the blend for this client, we make sure that it contains oils for treating back pain, oils for treating period pain, nervousness, and hypersensitivity, and oils for treating sleep disorders. It is possible that a particular oil will fill several of the required criteria. Similarly, we always pay attention to the hormonal system and the immune system.

To the same extent, we tailor the treatment method to the client. When treating back pains, for instance, we can opt to combine the essential oils with massage, which is the most common way of getting the oil into the body via the skin, and is, of course, of therapeutic value in and of itself for relaxing muscles and for treating problems of mobility. In contrast, if the person is suffering from insomnia, for example, our first choice of treatment might be an inhalation of an essential oil using an oil burner. We often combine several treatment methods in order to obtain the optimal results.

Client – a term that relates to a man or a woman (unless otherwise specified) who receives treatment from a practitioner, or who administers self-treatment using aromatherapy.

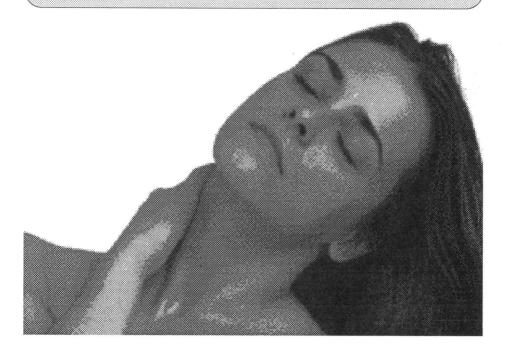

Selecting the oils

The cost of growing the raw materials for oil production may sometimes be very high. In some cases, several tons of petals from a particular flower are required in order to produce one liter of pure essential oil. The quality of the finished product is a function of how meticulous and professional the investment in the growth of the raw material – the plant – is. The process of growing the plant is extremely important, as is the harvesting or picking season, and of course, the fact that it is organically grown, without the use of insecticides and other chemical substances. Most of the professional oil manufacturers use organically grown plants. But the truth is that today, unfortunately, some of the raw materials have become rare or extinct, and therefore many of the oils have become extremely expensive. For this reason, many manufacturers have begun to sell diluted or synthetic substitutes, or impure blends.

When essential oils are used therapeutically in an oil burner, a compress, a bath, or a massage, only pure, high-quality oils are used. The "sensitivity" of the oils is so great and their quality so important that if we use a synthetic substitute or a diluted oil, it is impossible to achieve a result that comes anywhere near the result obtained from the use of pure essential oil. When blends are made in a less than professional manner, they are liable to contain synthetic components or a very low level of active ingredients. Therefore, when you purchase an essential oil, it is very important to buy it in a well-known and professional store only, and demand an oil from a reputable company. Many of the oils with exotic names such as "Opium," "Vanilla-Banana," and so forth, which are sold in New Age stores nowadays, must not be used for aromatherapy treatments under any circumstances. Those oils are meant for use in oil burners in order to create a pleasant odor in the house – nothing else. They are not therapeutic, and after they have been used in the burner, they tend to leave a powerful, unnatural odor that lingers even after the burner has been cleaned thoroughly. For this reason, it is not advisable to use a burner for aromatherapy treatments in which synthetic oils have been burned.

Remember that one of the properties of the oils can serve as a quality check: evaporation. Since the oils evaporate, they do not leave a stain. Exceptions to this rule are **rose** and **jasmine** oils, which may leave a stain. When you want to check whether an oil is pure, let a drop fall onto a piece of white cotton fabric or white paper. If the stain does not disappear after a few minutes, it means that the oil is not pure.

Rare oils, or oils that are extremely expensive to produce, tend to be very costly. For this reason, many imitations have appeared on the market. When you want to buy an oil of this type, you must check really carefully that the oil is pure and of high-quality.

Rose, chamomile, and **jasmine** oils are extremely expensive. Essential (absolute) oil produced from these plants is rare, and very costly. If you find one of these oils cheaply and from a company that is not known to be professional, it is not worth taking a chance.

Lavender oil is sometimes sold as a blend of **lavendine** – two wild strains of lavendula – and its quality is lower than that of pure **lavender** oil.

Louisa oil, which is considered a relatively rare and expensive oil, has many synthetic imitations, and the oil produced from Indian verbena or Spanish verbena may be sold as "Louisa" instead. These are not of the same quality as **louisa** oil. **Melissa** oil, too, is produced in small amounts, and various blends of citrus oils are often sold under the name of "melissa." Here, too, it is important to purchase the oil from a reliable source and from a well-known company. A similar problem exists with **neroli** oil. Genuine and original **neroli** is very expensive, and various blends of **petitgrain** oil with a tiny amount of **neroli** oil are often found on the market. When purchasing **rosewood** oil, too, it is important to ensure that it is not some synthetic blend that is being sold under the name of "rosewood." The price of this oil has risen sharply as a result of a shortage of raw materials – Brazilian rosewood trees, which are in danger of becoming extinct – and it is not easy to obtain genuine and pure oil. (Because of the difficult situation of rosewood trees, it is advisable to use other oils with similar properties.)

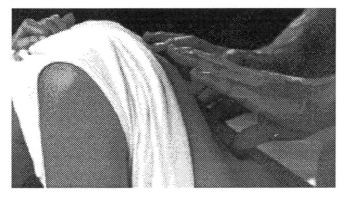

Essential oils – their proper care

After you have bought a professional and high-quality essential oil, it is very important to store it correctly.

As we said before, the oils are extremely sensitive, and they are greatly affected by weather conditions. At room temperature, the oils are in a liquid state. When they are chilled, they become more viscous, so if you choose to keep them in the refrigerator (which does extend their shelf-life), be sure to allow them to reach room temperature before you use them. Similarly, they are affected by humidity, so they should not be kept in a humid place. Remember not to leave the oil or the aromatic blend used for the bath in the bathroom, since humidity affects the quality of the oil. Light is another factor that affects the quality of the oil. Oils must not be left in sunlight, and it is important to store them in a dark and dry place (in a suitable closet, for instance). Heat is another factor that affects oils, so they must be removed from various sources of heat.

One of the biggest "enemies" of essential oils is oxygen. Oxidation causes the oil to spoil. Oil that is left in an open bottle will go off quickly, and its color and odor will change. For this reason, it is very important to keep the bottle tightly closed, and prevent the entry of oxygen as much as possible.

A bottle with an internal dropper is preferable, even though oils that come in a bottle with an external dropper keep well when they are properly stored. Similarly, the oil must be in a bottle made of dark glass, which prevents the penetration of light.

Most oils that are stored in optimal conditions will be good for about one year (citrus oils for about six months). Oil that is not stored in optimal conditions can go off even sooner.

How can you identify oil that has gone off?

When the oil you have purchased has changed color, its texture changes or becomes murky, its odor changes, its lid sticks, it becomes sticky or there are unidentifiable "things" floating in it – it means that the oil is off and must not be used!

Another property of the oils – one that we mentioned previously – is evaporation. In addition, all the oils dissolve in fat and in alcohol, in sugars and in salts, but they do not dissolve in water – they remain separate. Therefore, when using an oil in the bath, it is advisable to use one of the methods presented later on in order to ensure a better mixture of the oil with the bathwater.

Another point to remember when using oils is that the oils have their own life energy, which is important when using them in treatments. For this reason, they must be used gently, even when they are being mixed (that is, under no circumstances must the bottle be shaken hard in order to mix the oils), even when they are being dripped into the bathwater and mixed in. Using them roughly can damage them and adversely affect their quality.

Basic rules for preparing a blend of oils

One of the most important properties of oils is their synergism. Synergetic work means "team work," in which each oil in the blend influences the rest of the oils, and the sum of the components is greater than each one individually. For this reason, we do not use a blend containing more than four oils. There are oils that mix better with other oils, and complement them, but in principle, every oil can work with other oils. When the oils are combined, they "double their work." The combination of the components does better and more powerful work.

We must remember that this property (synergism) is one of the reasons why the use of a synthetic oil in a blend diminishes the power of the entire blend.

A combination of up to four oils in a blend enables us to strengthen the blend and balance it, to treat the client's entire range of problems, and obtain better results. When preparing a blend from several essential oils, it is important, of course, to ensure that the oils are suitable for treating all of the client's presented problems and disorders – but no less important to ensure that the blend is balanced in its odor and intensity.

There are various oils that stimulate and invigorate, and, in contrast, there are soothing oils. It is important that there be a balance between the soothing oils and the invigorating oils in the blend. Moreover, there are oils that are both soothing and invigorating.

There are stronger and weaker oils from the point of view of the dominance of their odor (each oil has its own note – low, medium and high). This must be calculated when preparing the blend. The best way to prepare the blend as regards balance and odors, especially when you are not very familiar with the particular odor of the oil, is to drip a tiny quantity of each oil in turn, and smell it, and then continue to drip. In this way, you will reach a balance in odor. Also, when preparing a blend from essential oils according to the formulas in this book, you must take into account the fact that oils of different manufacturers and different quality may differ in the intensity of their odor. Therefore, even when preparing the blend according to one of the given formulas, it is always advisable to drip a couple of drops of each oil in turn, smell the blend, check if its odor is balanced (that the odor of one oil does not dominate the entire blend), all the while sticking to the total number of drops (of all the essential oils together, since its dilution has been calculated according to the amount of carrier oil indicated) given in the book.

Toxicity of oils and allergies to oils

As with medicinal plants, so essential oils have varying degrees of toxicity, in accordance with their components and their active ingredients. There are essential oils with a higher degree of toxicity, and there are oils with a relatively low degree of toxicity. In any event, essential oils must not be used directly on the body unless they have been diluted. In rare cases, which are indicated in this book, especially for a localized area, it is possible to use a drop or two of undiluted essential oil, but in general, essential oils are used after being diluted in water, in carrier oil, in various creams, and so on. Exceptions to this are **lavender** oil and **tea tree** oil, which, because of their low toxicity, can be used directly on the body – *however, not for purposes of massage or for any purpose that requires a lot of oil for an extended time* – but only when in a small amount of essential oil (a few drops). Nevertheless, it is important to read the instructions on the bottle of **lavender** oil or **tea tree** oil. Moreover, you must check to see if the person is sensitive to these oils by doing a skin patch test – place a drop of undiluted oil on his wrist or behind his ear and wait a quarter-hour. If the person complains of a rash or a prickling sensation in the area, or if the area becomes red, or any other change occurs, the oil must not be used in its undiluted form. Among the warnings presented in this book are warnings about oils that must be tested on the client prior to working with them, even if they have been diluted in carrier oil. Similarly, the book indicates oils that have a high level of toxicity or that should not be used on a specific population group because of a certain property (pregnant women, infants, people who suffer from hypertension, and so on). There are also oils whose use is not recommended in general because of a high toxicity level.

Even if we use oils with a low level of toxicity, it is important to drink a lot of water after an aromatherapy treatment in order to flush the oil out of the body via the urine, after it has done its work.

Every six months or so, many practitioners take a break from the use of and treatment with essential oils after daily or frequent use of oils. Sometimes the break lasts for up to three months, sometimes only a few weeks – generally, each person senses how long he needs in order to "cleanse" himself. This point is important, since despite the superb action of the oils, and the fact that with correct, wise, and precise use of the oils, there is no risk or unpleasantness for the client, it is advisable to take a break after protracted and frequent use of oils in order to let the body continue its self-healing work unsupported for a time, and avoid the possibility of any kind of accumulation of substances that are found in the oils, even though they are harmless.

Another point that must be taken into account in aromatherapy is the possibility that the client may have an allergy to certain oils. As with any substance, organic or chemical, there may be people who are sensitive to oils, too (both carrier and essential oils). In general, the sensitivity is manifested in the skin by a rash, a prickling sensation, redness, and so on. The oils that may cause sensitivity are mainly the ones that belong to the citrus family, as well as the oils that contain limonene (**juniper** and **geranium**).

In all the professional literature concerning aromatherapy, it is stressed that the correct treatment with oils does not cause side effects, but there can be allergies and reactions.

What is a reaction?

A reaction is the body's response to aromatherapy (or to any other treatment – massage, reflexology, Bach flower remedies, and so on), since as a result of the treatment, the body undergoes a process of change that includes expelling toxins by releasing blockages and facilitating circulation. The process of expelling waste and toxins from the body is very important. In order to reach a state of balance, the waste must be expelled from the body, both on the physical and mental levels.

A reaction generally indicates a change in the body from a state of apparent balance to a state of genuine balance. Apparent balance is the body's way of becoming accustomed to an ongoing state of imbalance. For example, a smoker's body adapts itself to a cigarette; conversely, if a non-smoker smokes a cigarette, his body is likely to react by coughing in order to get rid of the foreign bodies in the cigarette, since his body is not used to these substances.

To the same extent, there are people who have been suffering from pain, such as back pain, for such a long time that they have gotten used to the pain and the poor state of their spine, or to the ongoing spasmodic state of their muscles. They are in a state of apparent balance and do not feel the pain consciously.

The reaction is not a side effect, like a reaction to medications, but it is the body's attempt to cleanse itself, to recover, and to restore its balance. When a combined treatment such as aromatherapy combined with reflexology or holistic massage is administered, the reactions are likely to be more significant. In order to reduce the reactions and the recovery crisis, the duration of the treatment is shortened and the treatments are administered less frequently.

As a rule, the reaction is welcome and wanted. It is better to go through it without medications and pills, and to let the body cope with its problems and expel the various toxins through tears, mucus, urine, and so on.

During a treatment with essential oils in combination with massage or reflexology, various reactions may occur. These could be yawning, smiling, a feeling of stress or fear, cramps, sweating, relaxation and pleasure, falling asleep, hunger, sexual arousal, talkativeness, a fierce urge to urinate, or extreme wakefulness. A reaction of exaggerated cold may attest to the client's low threshold of endurance and to an extreme inability to tolerate the treatment, so the treatment must be halted at this stage, and the client must be given a drink and covered.

More significant reactions can occur after the various treatments (again, mainly a treatment with essential oils in combination with reflexology or massage). In general, the reactions take place either in the organs of elimination – the digestive system, the urinary tract, the respiratory system, the skin (perspiration, blood, lymph) – or they can include excessive urination (one of the body's ways to get rid of its waste), skin rash, mucus (white, transparent), phlegm, coughing.

In rare cases, the following reactions can occur: nausea, diarrhea, excessive defecation, temporary constipation, sores, pimples, boils, mouth ulcers, dizziness, secretions from the eyes, the awakening of dormant inflammations (sinusitis, gingivitis, eye or intestinal inflammations, etc.), pains or symptoms in organs that were once ill or painful (back pain, asthma; an area that underwent surgery may suddenly feel sensitive and painful, and so on).

There can also be behavioral reactions – impatience, fatigue, openness, improved sleep patterns, restlessness, a feeling of exceptional calm, and so on. Generally, aromatherapy by itself, not in combination with massage, reflexology, or other techniques involving oil penetration, does not cause significant reactions (though these can occur). However, a common reaction is a "bizarre" sensation: headaches, light dizziness, various sensations in the digestive or respiratory system after smelling (via an oil burner, an inhalation or sniffing the bottle) one of the oils that has been matched with him. This frequently means that it is precisely that oil that is most suitable for the treatment of the client and evokes various sensations in him, because it is doing certain work on the client and reaching areas and systems in which there is an obvious state of imbalance.

However, in a case where the client feels a violent revulsion for the essential oil with which he is being treated, or experiences headaches or dizziness, it is a good idea to put the oil that is causing these sensations aside, treat the client with a different oil that has similar properties, and at a certain stage of the treatment, when the oils are changed, to try and check his feeling toward the particular oil once again. After a certain length of time of treatment, there may not be such a powerful reaction, and it will be possible to treat him with that oil.

While the reactions to aromatherapy are generally not significant, they may occur. A reaction may occur within two to three days of the treatment, or – particularly with massage – during the actual treatment. The reaction itself lasts *up to three days*. It can begin at the end of the treatment or the next day. A reaction that continues for more than three days may not be a reaction, but rather an illness to which the client has succumbed completely independently of the treatment. In this case, a physician must be consulted.

There are various factors that may intensify the reactions. For this reason, when the client arrives, he must be questioned as to his mental and family state, if he has undergone any changes recently (moving house, changes in eating habits), female changes, and so on). This is because when there are changes, the body is liable to be weaker and the reaction can be more significant. The following are factors that can intensify the reaction: a given mental state, time of year (there are people who are affected by the time of the year), personality structure, monthly period (because of hormonal changes), incubating a disease (at the beginning of the flu, a fever and cough – when there are already bacteria, it is advisable to administer a symptomatic treatment; however, it is not advisable to perform a holistic treatment with oils, including massage or reflexology, while any inflammation or acute disease is starting), nutritional habits (poor nutrition), low vitality (which can have a significant effect on the intensity of the reaction), environmental state (whether the client is stressed, calm), and so on.

As we said before, aromatherapy by itself generally does not cause serious reactions, but when it is combined with another kind of treatment, there could be significant reactions. It is very important to remember that the reaction is not a disease. It is welcome, and attests to changes that are occurring in the body and mind of the client as a result of the treatment. If the client experiences any kind of reaction, it is important to check whether it is indeed a reaction, and not a disease that developed independently of the treatment. (As you remember, a reaction continues for only a few days, and is nothing the client cannot endure or that endangers his health.) You must explain to him that he is having a reaction and there is no need to panic. (In an aromatherapy treatment in combination with reflexology, it is a good idea to explain the possibility of a reaction to the client right at the beginning of the treatment, since this effective and powerful combination is more likely to cause reactions.) It is important to support him right through the reaction, or in any change that he undergoes as a result of the treatment. Of course, the practitioner must not panic at the reactions, either, and if he feels any doubts, he should consult with a more experienced practitioner.

Substituting oils

Some practitioners change the blend of oils they prepare for a client about two to four months after beginning the treatment.

Exchanging the client's oils (in self-treatment as well) for other oils with similar properties has many advantages. It is important to let the oil perform its action for a certain length of time, but it is also very important to pay attention to the changes that occur in the client, which sometimes necessitate substituting one or more components – or even all the oils – in the blend.

This is how we prevent the client's body from "getting used to" the property of an oil that is likely to have an effect, introducing him instead to new oils with their own properties that provide a welcome variation in the treatment.

When substituting oils, it is not advisable to switch all four oils in the blend "in one go". Each time we decide to switch oils in the blend, it is advisable to switch only one or two at a time, and keep track of the developments.

For this reason, when substituting essential oils (or carrier oils), it is necessary to keep a meticulously written record of every client – and this is true for self-treatment as well.

The client's card contains:

The client's personal details, a record of the initial medical history-taking, (especially the primary problem, secondary problems, and possible causes), and treatment methods. In the record of the various blends, it is mandatory to indicate the type and amount of carrier oils and essential oils.

It is not enough to write down only the name of the oil – you must also write down the name of the manufacturer and preferably also the serial number (which appears on the products of certain companies). After every treatment or visit to the practitioner, it is mandatory to write down comments (efficacy of the treatment, changes of oil, and so on).

The principle is very simple: it is better to write down marginal and even "superfluous" details than to lose data.

2

Carrier oils

Because of the toxicity of the essential oils, they are not used in their undiluted form, but rather diluted in a carrier oil. In addition to lowering the level of toxicity in the blend, carrier oils enable the oil to be spread over the body and to penetrate it much more effectively. The advantage of a blend of carrier and essential oils lies in the fact that it permits a small quantity of essential oil to penetrate into a larger internal area. The carrier oils help the essential oils penetrate the body, and, in addition, slow down the absorption of the essential oil into the bloodstream (and thus, also, its exit from the body). In addition, carrier oils have their own properties, and they constitute an inseparable part of aromatherapy.

Carrier oils should always be cold pressed. They contain vitamins, minerals, and fatty acids. In contrast to essential oils, there is no limit to the number of carrier oils in a blend. It is possible to make a blend from a large number of oils, but the ease of working with the oil, its natural smell (which may be too strong or unpleasant for cosmetic use), and its degree of absorption in the body must be taken into account. Another property of carrier oils is that most of them can be taken orally, since they have a variety of healthful properties: they help prevent the accumulation of antioxidant fats, improve metabolism, improve peristalsis, promote the rise of the HDL ("good" cholesterol) level, and lower the LDL ("bad" cholesterol) level.

In external use, via the skin, the carrier oils add vitamins and minerals to the body, preserve skin moisture, improve skin elasticity, enrich the skin with fat, and nourish the skin with the vitamins, minerals, and fatty acids they contain.

Carrier or base oil is generally produced from three main parts of the plant:

1. From the seeds – carrier oils such as **sesame, grapeseed, wheatgerm**, and **sunflower**.

2. From the pits (with or without the fruit) – carrier oils such as **peach**, **apricot**, and **avocado**.

3. From the fruit – carrier oils that are produced from various nuts – **peanut**, **almond**, and **macadamia**.

Carrier oils contain various fatty acids. These acids, especially the essential fatty acids, have a far-reaching effect on the body. The fatty acids can be divided into three types:

1. Saturated fatty acids.

2. Monounsaturated fatty acids.

3. Polyunsaturated fatty acids.

The saturated fatty acids are found mostly in plants, such as oleic acid, for instance, which is present in a high concentration in **olive** oil.

Among the polyunsaturated fatty acids in the carrier oils, we can find linoleic acid, which is present in a high percentage in many oils, mainly in **wheatgerm** oil, **grapeseed** oil, **sweet almond** oil, **sunflower** oil, **soya bean** oil, and **rose-hip** oil. A by-product of linoleic acid, is present in **olive** oil and **peanut** oil. Linoleic acid is also present in **wheatgerm** oil, **grapeseed** oil, and **rose-hip** oil. Gamma-linoleic acid (GLA) is present in **olive** oil and **evening primrose** oil.

All the polyunsaturated fatty acids fulfill two main functions in the body: they participate in building the cell membrane, and serve as a raw material for important bodily compounds. The oils are effective because the skin cell membranes contain fat cells, so in order to preserve the elasticity of the skin, it is important to receive fatty acids either internally or externally.

Each of the fatty acids performs an important action in the body. Linoleic acid helps growth, prevents skin infections, lowers the cholesterol level in the blood, and serves as a raw material for an acid that is produced in the body from the linoleic acid, or comes directly from **peanut** and **olive** oil. It has anti-inflammatory properties. Linoleic acid is essential for the growth and development of the cells, the organs, and the body, and it is also anti-inflammatory.

A very important component that most of the cold-pressed oils contain is lecithin. Lecithin is produced in the liver, and it is a combination of choline and inozitol. Choline and inozitol have an important function in overseeing cholesterol and producing energy from the fats in the body. The importance of lecithin stems from the fact that it serves as a carrier for other substances, conveys fats in the blood, contributes to energy supply, and serves as an important component in the cells. The muscle that contains the biggest quantity of lecithin in the body is the heart muscle, and lecithin is important for its normal action. Lecithin's absorptive capacity in the body is good, and it increases the digestive and absorptive capacity of fats in the body, and can thus decrease the amount of fat particles that circulate in the body. It prevents them from accumulating on the cell walls and can dissolve both cholesterol and fats that have collected on the cell wall. It increases the digestive and absorptive capacity of cholesterol. Similarly, lecithin is an important component in the unsaturated fatty acids, and promotes good absorption of the vitamins that dissolve in fat (DEKA). Lecithin can be taken in capsule form, and is good for reducing cholesterol and triglycerides. It is slimming (it is a good idea to take a lecithin capsule after a heavy meal). One of the best ways to ensure a good, regular supply of lecithin to the body is to use cold-pressed oils, such as **olive** oil, **sesame** oil, regularly, and to add them as they are to various foods (that is, no cooking or frying).

Today, in the achievement-oriented and stressed-out West, the lack of lecithin is evident in many people. This is caused by situations of stress, fatigue, protracted over-exertion, and poor nutrition. For this reason, the use of carrier oils, whether externally via the skin, or internally (using suitable oils), helps, and is important for our health.

Lecithin can be found, as we said, in cold-pressed plant oils, but also in egg yolks, nuts, whole grains (especially wheat), soya, and in ox liver and heart. In all the foods that undergo refining processes (such as cooking and frying, for instance), the lecithin is destroyed. Another way of raising the lecithin level in the body is by regular physical activity.

There are many different types of carrier oils, and when we prepare an aromatherapy blend, we also take into account the properties of these oils in combination with the essential oils, in order to attain the best and effective result.

In general, when we prepare an aromatic blend, an important component in the blend of carrier oils is the one with the highest absorptive capacity in the skin, so that massaging the oils into the skin will be easy and effective. Therefore, oils that are "heavier" or that have a low absorptive capacity should constitute only about 20% of the blend. Moreover, we must be aware of the odor of the carrier oil – a carrier oil with a pungent odor is not suitable for a facial treatment, and sometimes not even for a general massage. At most, we might use a tiny amount of it in the blend.

Different types of carrier oils

Sweet almond oil

Only oil produced from sweet almonds should be used. **Almond** oil is one of the most common oils for aromatic use, since it is easily absorbed by the skin, almost completely odorless, pleasant to the touch, not expensive, and can be purchased easily in any store. **Almond** oil is rich in monounsaturated fatty acids.

Besides being pleasant to the touch and almost odorless – properties that make it superb for aromatherapy – **almond** oil also softens the skin, serves as a substitute for facial cleansing oil, is suitable for all skin types, and is recommended for the treatment of oily skin. In the treatment of oily skin, **sweet almond** oil slightly dries the skin by removing the unwanted fatty layer. In general, **almond** oil serves as a base for the heavy carrier oils and dilutes them. It must be remembered that this oil may dry out sensitive or very dry skin. The oil's absorption is very good, and it is considered to be a "light" oil.

Grapeseed oil

Grapeseed oil is produced from the seeds of grapes, and, like **sweet almond** oil, is also popular because of its rapid absorption into the body, its lack of odor, its low price, and its availability.

Grapeseed oil contains saturated fatty acids, and linoleic acid, and contains a very high percentage of GLA. It also contains vitamin E.

Grapeseed oil, which is gentle and pleasant to the touch, is absorbed in the body well, shrinks and knits tissues, and is good for treating all the problems that stem from dry skin – eczema, allergies, rashes, and so on.

Apricot kernel oil

Apricot kernel oil is considered to be a luxury oil, and is very common in facial and cosmetic treatments. It has a high absorptive capacity in the skin, and permeates it well. It is very convenient to use and pleasant to the touch. **Apricot kernel** oil is very suitable for treating dry skin, since it helps preserve the skin's moisture and improves its elasticity. It is rich in vitamin A.

Peach kernel oil

Peach kernel oil is considered to be a luxury oil (it is not always available, since it is mainly imported from England). This oil is very similar in its properties and use to **apricot kernel** oil. It is considered to be excellent for facial and cosmetic treatments, but costs more than **apricot kernel** oil. Its absorptive capacity is very good, and it is convenient to use and pleasant to the touch.

Evening primrose oil

This oil is produced from the yellow flowers of the evening primrose, which opens only at night. It is thought to be a superb oil for cosmetic treatments. It contains gamma-linoleic acid (GLA) and prostaglandins (PGE), which constitute a raw material in the body for hormones and neurotransmitters.

Evening primrose oil is good for maintaining blood vessels, for regulating blood pressure, for dilating blood vessels, and for preventing thromboses. It helps regulate cholesterol and insulin levels, produce T-lymphocytes, prevent the synthesis of cholesterol, and prevent inflammatory processes and allergies. In addition, the oil helps prevent allergies in the body, so it is used in the treatment of inflamed, sensitive, and allergic skin. Moreover, it improves the regeneration of skin cells, which makes it a wonderful oil for treating damaged, neglected, tired, and aging skin. Some people use it in the treatment of alcoholics in order to prevent damage to the liver and other damage caused by alcoholism. It may help alcoholics kick the habit. It is not cheap, and is used for facial and cosmetic treatments in aromatherapy.

Rose-hip oil

Rose-hip oil is generally sold in small quantities and is not cheap. The best type comes from Chile. **Rose-hip** oil contains linoleic acid. It has a good absorptive capacity in the skin, softens the skin, is anti-inflammatory, promotes blood circulation, and is very common in the treatment of wrinkles and stretch marks.

Passionflower oil

Passionflower oil is used in facial and cosmetic treatments. It contains a large quantity of linoleic acid, contributes to the improvement of the appearance of the skin, and generally a few drops of it are dripped into a blend of other carrier oils.

Gold-of-pleasure oil

This is a luxury cosmetic oil that is produced from the camelina plant. It is rich in linoleic acid, and is used in cosmetic treatments in order to improve the appearance of the skin.

Borage oil

This pleasant oil is generally used in cosmetic and facial treatments, when a few drops of it are dripped into a blend of other carrier oils, such as **almond** oil or **grapeseed** oil. Since it contains gamma-linoleic acid, it is very helpful in lowering the level of sensitivity and allergy of sensitive skin. In addition, it helps the regeneration of the skin cells. It is very suitable for treating sensitive skin or skin that is inflamed as a result of allergies, and for treating aging or "tired" skin.

Calendula (Marigold) oil

When purchasing **calendula** oil, make sure to check that the oil really is pure and cold-pressed. Of course, we are not talking about cooking oil. **Calendula** oil is used in various cosmetic treatments, especially for stretch marks and cracked skin, and a small quantity of it can be added to a blend of other carrier oils.

Cherry kernel oil

This carrier oil is a wonderful cosmetic oil. A few drops of it can be dripped into the blend in order to enhance the activities of the oils in improving the appearance of the skin and its elasticity. It contains a high level of linoleic acid, is absorbed into the skin well, and is considered to be a luxury oil.

Sesame oil

Sesame oil is used for seasoning salads and other foods, and is recommended for internal use. It is a good idea to substitute **sesame** oil, with its subtle and interesting flavor, for commercial brands of salad dressing.

Sesame oil is rich in minerals, especially calcium, magnesium, phosphorus, iron, and lecithin, as well as vitamin E and the vitamin B complex. As we said before, this oil is recommended for internal use. When used in this way, it enriches the blood by raising the level of the red blood corpuscles. It is highly recommended for children with anemia (about 20 drops of **sesame** oil daily for a month) and for pregnant women with an iron problem (a tablespoon of **sesame** oil daily). Moreover, it is good for activating the spleen (which is an important partner in the action of the immune system) enhances liver and gallbladder function, and constitutes a good source of vegetable protein.

In aromatherapy, we mainly focus on the oil's properties when used externally (via massage and application to the skin). **Sesame** oil preserves the skin's moisture, improves its elasticity, helps lighten the skin (spots on the surface of the skin and so on), is suitable for every skin type, possesses an element of protection, thus protecting the skin from the sun, and is considered to be a very energetic oil that is effective in treating people who suffer from the cold. The oil's rapid absorption makes it suitable for many facial and body treatments. Having said that, it has a conspicuous odor, and is generally not used as a basic carrier oil or as the only carrier oil in a blend.

Avocado oil

Avocado oil is obtained from the ripe fruits of the avocado tree. It is rich in fatty acids, and contains saturated fatty acids, a large quantity of oleic acid (which helps lower blood pressure, sclerosis of the arteries, and heart diseases), and linoleic acid. Moreover, it contains a range of oil-soluble vitamins – E, A, and D, as well as vitamin C.

The oil of **avocado kernels** penetrates the skin well, softens it, helps make it pliant – mainly via its beneficial action on the collagen fibers in the connective tissue, and for this reason is good for the treatment of dry, wrinkled, or neglected skin. By using this oil, it is possible to rehabilitate skin that has lost its pliancy after a disease that has affected the skin, as a result of dehydration, and so on. **Avocado** oil is absorbed slowly, and therefore it should constitute no more than 20% of a blend.

Sunflower oil

Sunflower oil is produced from sunflower seeds, and it is important to mention that we are talking about the cold-pressed oil and not the common cooking oil. **Sunflower** oil contains saturated fatty acids and polyunsaturated fatty acids, the greater portion of which is linoleic acid. Moreover, it contains the minerals calcium, zinc, potassium, iron, and phosphorus, as well as the vitamin B complex and a large quantity of vitamin E.

Cold-pressed **sunflower** oil is highly recommended for internal use because of its high percentage of unsaturated fatty acids, which help lower the cholesterol level.

This oil is also a diuretic and cleanses the body. It is good for building teeth and bones in children (because of its calcium content).

When used externally, the oil is absorbed well in the skin. It is good for facial treatments (because it contains zinc, a very important mineral for facial skin), acne, sores that do not heal, and so on.

Wheatgerm oil

Wheatgerm oil constitutes an important supplement to every aromatic blend, both because of its high mineral and vitamin content and because of its property of protecting the blend from oxidation, thus helping to increase the life span of the aromatic blend and maintain its quality. Because it is a thick, heavy oil, it should not constitute more than 20% of a blend.

Wheatgerm oil contains saturated fatty acids, of which about half is linoleic acid. It contains the minerals zinc, iron, potassium, magnesium, and phosphorus, the vitamins B1, B2, B5, B6, and a very large quantity of vitamin E, which is an extremely important antioxidant.

When used internally, **wheatgerm** oil lowers the cholesterol level in the blood, prevents sclerosis of the arteries, is good for preventing heart diseases and for purifying the blood, and is important for neutralizing free radicals. The oil helps in building muscles and bones in children. Moreover, it is good for digestive problems and helps the normal development of the blood vessels. For this reason, it is highly recommended to take the oil orally in cases of various blood vessel diseases.

When used externally, **wheatgerm** oil is good for allergic conditions, eczema, skin blisters, burns, and psoriasis. *Remember that this oil must not be used when treating people with celiac disease.*

Wheatgerm oil is very heavy and is absorbed into the skin slowly, so that when used externally, it must always be combined with a lighter and more rapidly absorbed carrier oil (such as **almond** oil, **grapeseed** oil, and so on).

Olive oil

Olive oil, which is very well known, is a wonderful oil for both internal and external use. Since it contains a relatively low level of saturated fatty acids, it is very suitable for internal use, and it contains many saturated fatty acids.

When used internally, the presence of linoleic acid causes the oil to be less sensitive to oxygenation, and thus lowers the chances of the formation of free radicals, which in turn slows down the aging process. **Olive** oil helps lower the level of LDL ("bad" cholesterol), improves blood flow, helps lower blood pressure by dilating the blood vessels, prevents and inhibits heart disorders, helps improve the absorption and maintenance of the calcium level in the bones, catalyzes and enriches the secretion of gall (thus also helping to break down the fats better), helps break down and prevent gallstones, is good in cases of heartburn and peptic ulcers, soothes coughs, and is recommended for nursing mothers (a teaspoon of olive oil a day). Moreover, it is wonderful for the treatment of constipation when taken internally. (For treating constipation, one tablespoon of olive oil in half a glass of warm water should be taken in the morning, on an empty stomach. This blend is excellent for stimulating the gallbladder and the liver and for alleviating constipation.)

When used externally, too, **olive** oil has extremely important properties. It is an analgesic oil, which means that it is suitable for treating pains in general, as well as pains in the joints and bones, and pains resulting from sprains and fractures. It is good for various skin problems (since it contains GLA), for treating the hair, earache, psoriasis, and skin inflammations.

Despite its marvelous properties, we are faced with several problems regarding the use of **olive** oil in aromatic blends. Its smell is very dominant, which means that it is not suitable for facial treatments (though there are people who like the smell very much); it is very viscous and heavy, and as a result of its heaviness, is absorbed very slowly in the skin. Because of these properties, it must always be mixed with one of the lighter carrier oils, and it should not constitute more than 20% of a blend.

Soya oil

Cold-pressed **soya** oil (not the kind that is used for cooking) is obtained from soya beans. It is rich in polyunsaturated fatty acids and is cholesterol-free. It contains linoleic acid, oleic acid, and saturated fatty acids. It is also rich in proteins.

When used externally, **soya** oil has several disadvantages that discourage its use in facial treatments and massage. The main one is its unpleasant odor. Moreover, it tends to spoil quickly. Since it helps with menopausal problems and PMS, it should be taken orally by adding it to salads and cold foods (in order not to damage its qualities by cooking or frying).

Jojoba oil

Jojoba oil, which is produced from the beans of the jojoba plant, is a heavy oil, reminiscent of wax, and for this reason is used in the manufacture of various ointments instead of glycerin. When used externally, it has important qualities: besides antibacterial properties, it has anti-inflammatory properties, which means that it is good for treating skin and joint inflammations. As a rule, this oil is superb for treating all inflammatory conditions. Moreover, it is good for the digestive system, helps the normal development of the blood vessels, is an antioxidant, reduces the viscosity of the blood, and is good for treating eczema. **Jojoba** oil is widely used in cosmetic treatments and in the treatment of dry, wrinkled, and aging skin, because of its effective action in preventing the evaporation of water from the skin. Also, it protects the skin against UV rays.

Since it is very heavy and penetrates right down into the deep tissues, there is a danger of oil accumulation, so it should not constitute more than 30% of the blend. Another carrier oil must be added, such as **almond** oil, **sesame** oil, and so on. The absorption of **jojoba** oil is slow, and that is another reason that prevents us from using a higher percentage of it in a blend of carrier oils.

Peanut (ground nut) oil

In its original form, **peanut** oil is not absorbed quickly in the body – on the contrary, it has a relatively low absorptive capacity. Sometimes, it is possible to purchase this oil already mixed with another carrier oil such as **almond** oil. **Peanut** oil oils the epidermis and thus prevents the skin from splitting and prevents the appearance of scales. It can constitute up to 30% of a blend.

Coconut oil

Coconut oil is produced from the covering of the nut itself. It is a semi-solid oil that solidifies in the cold. **Coconut** oil contains a very high percentage of saturated fatty acids, which means that it is less effective for treatment and is therefore not recommended for the skin or for taking orally. This oil is used in the manufacture of chocolate and soap. Its main use in aromatherapy is as a covering and protection for the hair, when spread only on the hair and not on the scalp. In the winter, the oil tends to freeze, which means that it has to be warmed up in a saucepan containing hot (but not boiling) water, and it must be remembered that it does not blend well with other plant oils. Its main use is for preparing hair masks for protecting the hair.

Palm oil

This oil is obtained from the fruit of the palm tree. It contains saturated fatty acids and linoleic acid. It is a very heavy oil, with properties similar to those of **coconut** oil. In the food industry it is used for the manufacture of margarine, sweets, soaps, and the inner covering of cans. This oil also does not blend well with other plant oils, tends to solidify in the winter, and has to be warmed up before use (in the same way as **coconut** oil). It is not suitable for external use on the skin, but is good for the hair in the form of a mask (just for the hair, not the scalp), and is even preferable to **coconut** oil.

Preparing a blend with carrier oils and essential oils

After we have chosen the suitable carrier and essential oils that are effective in treating the problem at hand, we can begin to prepare the blend. The rules for preparing a blend of essential and carrier oils vary according to the age of the client and his level of vitality.

For the adult client (in principle from age 12, unless the youngster is thin, small, or frail for his/her age; in that case, he/she is considered a child), for every 2 cc (ml) of carrier oil, we use one drop of essential oil. That is, the drops of essential oil constitute half of the number of cc (ml) of the carrier oils. For instance, for a quantity of 40 cc of carrier oil, we use 20 drops of essential oil. If the adult client is weak, post-illness, very thin, or has a low level of vitality, we use a smaller quantity of essential oils. The same goes for treating the elderly, who sometimes have to be treated with the amounts that are used for treating big children (in accordance with their state of health and strength). The measure that is used in the treatment of an adult is considered to be a "whole" unit, and constitutes the yardstick for preparing a blend for younger clients.

For big children, from eight to twelve (again, it is important to pay attention to whether the child is big or small for his age, and then act accordingly), we use *half* the amount of essential oil as we do for adults. In other words, if we used 20 drops of essential oil to 40 cc of carrier oil, here we use 10 drops of essential oil to 40 cc of carrier oil.

When treating small children, from three to six or seven, we use *a quarter* of the "whole" amount of essential oil. In other words, if we use 40 cc of carrier oil, we only use five drops of essential oil.

When treating infants up to age two, we must be extremely alert to the infant's condition and strength. In principle, we use *an eighth or less* of the amount of essential oil. In other words, if we use 40 cc of carrier oil, we will use only two drops of essential oil. In the case of a very young or weak infant, we add more carrier oil to the blend, just to make sure. The infants' bodies are more delicate, so the oils are absorbed into their bodies very quickly, and their action is also faster than with adults. Children and infants react well to treatment with essential oils, and results are often achieved extremely fast.

In any event, one of the rules we must remember when preparing a blend of essential oils and carrier oils is *not to mix* more than 20 drops of essential oil into the carrier oil, even if we have exceeded the amount of 40 cc carrier oil and are using 50 or 60 cc.

The limit is 20 drops of aromatherapy oils in the blend for a single client in every form of treatment.

> *The aromatherapy treatments for certain diseases and problems that are presented in this book derive from the experience of the authors, and are based on actual cases. Occasionally, due to various considerations (the seriousness of the problem, the physical strength of the client, the use of safe and "easily effective" aromatherapy oils, the use of pure but "diluted" aromatherapy oils produced by particular companies, and so on), the practitioners chose to increase the amount of essential oil in the mixture.*
>
> *An experienced practitioner can deviate from the "no more than 20 drops" limit mentioned above. Even so, he has to weigh his decision very carefully.*
>
> *The beginner practitioner would do well to observe the limit – even in the few cases in which, in the description of the case, the experienced practitioner decided to act differently.*

3

Methods of treatment

The methods of using essential oils in treatments are many and varied, and are suitable for a vast range of physical and emotional problems.

The two most common methods of treatment are massage (in which the oil enters the body through the skin) and treatment with a burner, which mainly affects emotional conditions (the oil reaches the body's tissues via the respiratory system).

Other common methods of using essential oils in treatments are various baths, hot and cold compresses, reflexology massages, vaginal douches, application to the skin, and inhalation.

In some cases, we will use several of the methods of treatment together in order to achieve optimal results, but in treatments that are considered "big" (that is, very significant in the way they affect the body), we will not perform two of them on the same day. In other words, treatments with massage, a bath, and reflexology using essential oils will not all be administered on one day.

Moreover, it is not advisable to administer reflexology or massage on consecutive days, but these treatments can be administered alternately with bath treatments (a massage one day, a bath one day). This is a particularly therapeutic combination, and is used at the beginning of aromatherapy and for treating extreme cases. It must not continue for a long time (up to two weeks, and then the frequency of the treatments must be reduced).

Experienced professional practitioners determine the duration and the frequency of the treatments in accordance with the individual client's condition and the changes that occur in his condition as a result of aromatherapy.

Massage

Massage is a common and popular method of getting the essential oils to penetrate the body via the skin. Massage is performed using a blend of carrier oil and essential oils, and has many advantages, both on its own and when combined with aromatherapy. Massage combines touch, which itself is therapeutic – both physically and mentally – with the action of the oils. The penetration of the oil makes the massage more effective, and the massage itself causes the oils to penetrate the skin better. In addition, massage stimulates the flow of blood and lymph, and the circulatory system, activates the immune system, and invigorates, thus stimulating all the body's systems. Massage helps cleanse the body of waste and toxins, and leads to improved excretion of waste from the body. In cases of various pains, especially muscular pains, the relief afforded by massage with essential oils is very significant, as it is in conditions that require the reduction of swelling and congestion. Massage induces general tranquillity and repose, and, in accordance with the use of oils, can even help the person feel more alert and energetic. On the mental plane, massage helps open energetic blockages, lower mental stress, release mental reactions, and raise energy levels and vitality.

There are different types of massage. Among the most common is Swedish massage, which is divided into two: (a) effleurage movements, which are slow and rhythmic, and consist of spreading movements and primal touch, and encompass the body. The greater the pressure exerted in this movement, the greater its effect on the muscles and blood vessels. The weaker the pressure exerted, the greater its effect on the nerves; (b) petrissage movements, which are kneading movements that are performed with the whole palm and the fingers.

Neuromuscular massage, which is exactly what its name suggests, works on the muscles and the nerves and is performed on both sides of the spine (but not on the spine itself!). This massage is meant to release the muscles, the tendons, the connective tissues, and the nerves, and they are released by applying pressure on the tissues and on certain areas on the back. When you press on a nerve, all the organs and areas connected to this nerve are affected.

Massage that is combined with pressure movements – Shiatsu – on pressure points, works on the meridians, and when we use it, we activate the body's meridians.

Massage techniques

1. Effleurage

Effleurage movements are slow, rhythmic movements, kind of light brush-strokes. To perform these movements, we mostly use the surface of the palm.

This movement is very suitable for the initial touch, and it can be done very softly, or much more closely to the body, so that the sliding is stronger and felt more. When effleurage is performed at the beginning of the massage, we should start with light movements. When using massage oils, effleurage is suitable for the initial spreading of the oil. Using effleurage, it is possible to perform movements that encompass the body, and provide a feeling of warmth, protection, and tranquillity. It can be used on the back, and on the arms; both hands can be used on each side of the client's arm, sliding them, and applying the appropriate amount of pressure. The legs can be treated in the same way. On the back and chest, large, encompassing movements should be used. It is important to remember to maintain the same pressure throughout the movement, when it is applied to a large surface, like the back. Performing this movement on the sides of the back gives the client a wonderful feeling.

It is also important to remember that the fingers should not be too spread out, in order not to lose energy and power while performing the movement. In effleurage, the greater the pressure, the more effect it has on the muscles and the blood vessels. The weaker the pressure, the greater the effect on the nerves (and the less the effect on the muscles and blood vessels). Some masseurs are in the habit of beginning and ending the massage with a few effleurage movements, so as to create a warm and pleasant feeling of closing the circle, and preserving the results that were achieved during the massage.

2. Kneading

The kneading movements are reminiscent of kneading bread. They are performed by using the palm and the fingers, grasping the correct amount of tissues with the hand and fingers, so as not to pinch the skin. As opposed to effleurage, it is a very vigorous movement. Of course, it can be performed gently, or with greater pressure.

Too much oil applied to the area can impair the movement. Kneading releases the tissues, invigorates the blood, and works well with the muscles.

Kneading is performed very gently, mainly on the surface of the abdomen, and on the buttocks, the arms and the legs (on the back, a variation of this movement, called "squeezing," or petrissage, is performed), pulling the thumb in an inward direction, and the rest of the fingers, using the entire palm, in an outward direction. This is one of the most pleasant and releasing movements for the shoulders, in order to release contractions and pain.

3. Squeezing (petrissage)

The petrissage movement, like effleurage, is also one of the basic movements – especially in Swedish massage and deep tissue massage. This is a most effective movement for releasing tensions and pressures in the tissues, nerves, and muscles, but a certain amount of practice is required in order to perform it optimally. To perform the movement, we gently grasp the skin between the thumb and the rest of the fingers. It is better to begin it from the top and go downward, and after gaining experience and a good and correct feeling in the hands, it is possible to change the directions, using different variations, and combining petrissage with other massage techniques.

After grasping the skin between the thumb and the fingers, we squeeze it gently and let it go, using a light revolving movement beneath the fingers. This is a marvelous movement to perform on the back, and initially, it is a good idea to perform it mainly in that area, until the feeling in the hands improves. After a little experience, it can be performed on the upper part of the arm as well, and on the back of the thighs and the calves. (Not everyone can tolerate this movement on these areas of the body.) We must pay attention to how the client feels about this movement.

It is important for this movement to be smooth; it begins at a particular point, and continues downward or upward along the whole surface, which effectively loosens tightness.

4. Revolving

The revolving movement is used mainly in physiotherapy. It is a movement by means of which we gently, freely, and smoothly turn the joints of the body. This movement is performed on the shoulders, knees, ankles, neck, and elbows. It is important to remember to support the joint firmly. When we feel that the area is very stiff and painful, we perform the movement very gently and slowly. To complete the release, we can perform it faster and more lightly.

To demonstrate, think of the movements performed by a person who wants to loosen his shoulders; he revolves them a few times in one direction, and then in the other.

It is important to remember that we do not massage an injured or diseased joint. This movement must not be performed by force! "Beginner" masseurs must be doubly cautious when applying it.

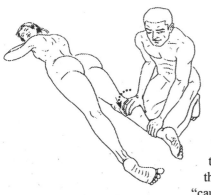

5. Rolling

The rolling movement is a soft and releasing movement, which is applied on a relatively large surface of the body. The rolling is performed using the whole palm and all the fingers. Its aim is to move and rock relatively large areas simultaneously, and it gives a pleasant movement of relaxing and loosening the tissues. The rolling movement is very suitable for treating the thighs, from the top down, on the back part of the calves (which are sometimes too stiff and "caught" to have petrissage performed on them), on the upper part of the arms, and on the buttocks. Since we can perform this movement very softly, and regulate its intensity, we should use it in order to work on areas that are too stiff to be treated by stronger movements, such as petrissage, or to "prepare the groundwork" for massage, preferably after performing a few circular and enveloping effleurage movements.

6. Rubbing-Pulling

The rubbing-pulling movement can be used at the beginning of the massage, for preparing the body, using long, slow movements, or during the massage, for invigorating the blood (in more dynamic movements). With rubbing-pulling movements, we pass one hand, or both, over the body in a rubbing movement, while applying a little pressure. In general, the movements are performed vertically, but they can also be performed horizontally (at the sides of the back, for instance, while standing at the client's side). The slower and "rounder" the movement, the more relaxation and tranquillity it will provide. The faster and more vigorous it is, resembling actual rubbing, the more effective it will be in invigorating the blood. It is accepted practice to perform the movement on the back, on the sides of the back, and on the ribs (since it is not a deep movement, it can be applied to the ribs, as it does not hurt, but stimulates or soothes, according to the speed of the movement), on the chest, the arms, and the legs. When we perform the movement on the arms or legs, we can pull and rub with one hand, and hold onto the leg or hand with the other for support.

7. Turning-rubbing

This is one of the most pleasant and soothing movements in massage. To perform the turning-rubbing technique, we mainly use the pads of our fingers, although skilled masseurs are likely to discover that they can perform this movement on larger surfaces using the pad of the palm as well. We use the soft parts of the hand – the pads of the hands and the pads of the fingers. This movement can thus be applied to parts of the face, to the temples (using the fingers – marvelous!), with small, circular movements on parts of the head – while sliding into the shampooing movement that will be described later, on the neck, the elbows, the knees, and the ankles. By paying a lot of attention when performing these movements, and by focusing on the fingertips that move in circular movements, both the practitioner and the client simultaneously are likely to experience a wonderful sensation.
There is some importance to the direction of the circle, whether clockwise or anti-clockwise, and a practitioner who feels an intuitive "need" to apply the movement to a particular area in a particular direction should heed his inner feelings and act accordingly. These movements have a unique effect on the mind, especially when the massage is gentle and considerate.

8. Pulling pressure

In the pulling pressure movement we place both palms on the client's back. We should start from the center of the back, when we place both palms horizontally (across the width of the client's back, near each other), with the inner part of the palm, the hollow, over the vertebra region, so that no pressure is exerted on them. We should stand at the client's side while performing the movement. In a vigorous and steady manner, we pull each palm in the opposite direction – one upward, all the way toward the shoulders, and the other downward, in the direction of the curve of the buttocks. The pulling movement must be clear-cut and steady, but not painful, out of sensitivity to the client's body.

We can also perform the movement from the upper part of the thighs (where they begin) to the tip of the toes, but here we perform the pulling in a downward direction only.

Both hands can be placed gently on either side of the inner part of the knee (the hollow; not right on it, since it is a delicate area), with one hand pulling in the direction of the calf, and the other in the direction of the thigh, in a stretching movement, while they slide over those parts. This movement creates a feeling of stretching the skin and the tissues, and is likely to be very effective in relieving pain, especially after protracted physical activity.

We also use pulling pressure movements when massaging the face. Here we perform them delicately, steadily, and slowly with the fingers, on both sides of the client's forehead, pulling toward the sides of the head; using almost the full length of the forefinger on each side of the bridge of the nose, pulling gently in the direction of the cheeks; and using the pads of the fingers on the eyebrows, pulling in the direction of the temples. When massaging the face, the movements are performed gently and slowly.

9. Shaking

Shaking movements are movements that are performed in a steady and dynamic way using both hands. They are fast movements, which can be performed on the upper part of the back, on the thighs, and on the buttocks. They are very pleasant, releasing, and dynamic. In a therapeutic massage, we try to perform the movements in the area of the buttocks and the thighs inward, in order to prevent any possible unpleasant feeling on the part of the client in these sensitive areas. (In contrast, in a sexually arousing and erotic massage, movements that are performed in an outward direction are likely to arouse the person sexually because they have a stimulating effect on the nerves in the thigh, buttock, and groin regions). In a therapeutic massage, we perform these movements very dynamically and at a high speed. In an erotic massage, they can be performed more slowly, so that they can work more on the nerves.

10. Shampooing

The shampooing movement, which is performed on the scalp, is familiar to many people from the beauty salon or the barber shop. Of course, during massage, we do not perform these movements quickly or perfunctorily, but slowly, with a good instinct for the stiff areas of the client's scalp. To perform the movement, we have to stand, or sit (more comfortable from the point of view of height) behind the client's head, when he is lying on his back with his head protruding slightly from the bed.

The movement is performed using the fingers and the pads of the hands. We gently ease our fingers between the client's strands of hair, preferably starting from the bottom – from the place where the head joins the neck, and we begin to rub and massage the delicate tissue of the scalp with soft, circular movements. A little bit of pressure can be applied, but we must remember to support the client's head with the pads of our palms, while the fingers perform the shampooing movement. It is possible to perform vigorous movements that stimulate, invigorate, and increase alertness.

Soft, slow, rhythmical movements induce a state of deep relaxation (in certain cases, a state of alpha waves). Some people use this movement before a guided visualization, for example, because of the deep relaxation it induces.

It is a wonderful way of releasing the many tensions that concentrate in the region of the head.

11. Neuromuscular massage on both sides of the spinal column

This massage aims to release the muscles, the tendons, the connective tissue, and the nerves. It is performed mainly by the fingers, but also by the pads of the hands, and it must be performed extremely carefully. When the practitioner is experienced, he can also find the specific points along the spinal column that are stiff. We begin from the top of the spinal column – under no circumstances along the spinal column itself, but on each side. At the beginning of the massage, when using the fingers, and the body is not yet relaxed and loose enough, the movements must be performed with the fingers with extreme gentleness; pressure can be used, but it must be gentle pressure that is not too invasive, because we will probably encounter many stiff points on our way, and penetrating them too deeply with our fingers is liable to hurt the client.

After we have performed this technique several times, or feel that the muscles on both sides of the spinal column are looser, we can use our fingers to penetrate a bit into the places where we felt some stiffness. The penetration is performed by placing the pad of the finger on the point, and applying a steady, slow pressure inward for a number of seconds.

In the same slow manner in which we entered the tissue, we also leave it.

To perform this technique, a great deal of sensitivity in the hands is required, as well as an ability to feel the client's body in the correct way. Beginner masseurs must first perform the movements with extreme gentleness, more in order to learn than to loosen muscles, until they learn how to perform this technique correctly without hurting the client. By using this technique, we can release muscles, connective tissues, and nerves very successfully. We must remember that when we press on a nerve, we affect all the organs and areas it serves. An inexperienced masseur – especially an amateur – must not begin with deep, penetrative finger work. He can simply pull his fingers slowly along the spinal column in order to release the connective tissue, the muscles, and the nerves that are nearer the surface.

12. Tapping/Slapping/Chopping

In the tapping movements, the fingertips tap and drum on the body quickly, one after the other. This is a percussive movement, and the fingers must be spread like a rake in order to perform it and "drum" gently on the body. This movement greatly stimulates the nerve endings and invigorates the blood flow. It is performed on the whole posterior side of the body, also concentrating on the area between the shoulder joint and the chest (the area below the clavicle, in the direction of the shoulder). These movements can be performed extremely gently (only on a healthy person) on the chest region as well, in order to stimulate the thymus gland and ease congestion, and to release nervous and muscle tension in the chest.

In the "drum" movements, we curve our hands and drum with them, one at a time, creating a hollow sound.

The slapping movements are performed on the posterior side of the patient's body quickly and alternately. To perform the movements, we flatten our hands, just like when giving a slap, but of course, we perform the movement softly, albeit with determination. These movements invigorate the blood capillaries near the surface of the skin, and the nerves that are located in the topmost layer of the skin, and cause an increase in the sensations of the skin.

We use the chopping movement on the outer side of the hands (from the outer side of the pinkie to the outer side of the pad of the palm). These dynamic and fast movements are similar in form to karate chops, but are gentler, of course. The movements accelerate the blood flow, and are wonderful for the circulation. After a few minutes of "drumming" using these fast movements, the client will feel warmth and vigor, as well as tranquillity and relaxed muscles.

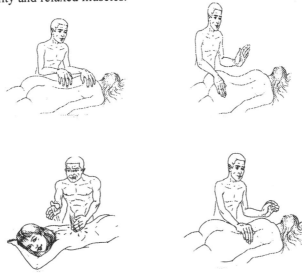

Since massage with essential oils is a relatively "powerful" treatment, there are cases in which it cannot be used. The counter-indications of massage include the following cases:

Viral diseases/infections at the acute stage – massage is liable to increase the symptoms and make them more extreme, and may even spread the infection to other areas of the body;

Cases in which there is a high fever;

Bruises (here we only apply the oil without massaging it into the skin);

Open sores (when treating sores, we drip suitable oils onto the specific area – refer to the section on first aid for more details);

Burns (these are also given specific treatment with essential oils, as described in the section on first aid);

All heart diseases, and also stages of recuperation after a heart disease or heart surgery;

Acute diseases involving medications, as well as clients who take "cocktails" of medications (as in certain cases of diabetes, AIDS, and so on), since the massage will cause the medications to be expelled from the body much more quickly than usual (these cases are not given baths, either);

Internal surgery – for the first three months following the surgery, massage is not given; afterwards, treatment by gentle application is administered (gentle, localized application is also possible beforehand, when treating other organs, but not the area of surgery);

Cancer cases – these require a physician's authorization;

Inflamed, congested, and swollen areas, such as a sprain or a fracture;

Cases of sharp inflammation of the veins and inflamed varicose veins. Varicose veins are treated only with very gentle and localized massage – see the section that deals with this topic).

Massage is highly recommended for relief and release in cases of spinal tension – by means of neuromuscular work (that is, work on the nerves that extend from the spine into the body), since it achieves excellent results.

Duration of a massage treatment

A massage treatment for adults can last for an hour and even an hour and a quarter. A massage treatment for big children (from seven or eight to twelve) can last for a half-hour, but we must note whether the child is big or small for his age, and decide on the duration of the treatment accordingly. For instance, a 12-year-old child with the physical build of a 14-year-old can undergo a massage treatment for up to three-quarters of an hour. Conversely, an eight-year-old child with the physical build and development of a six-year-old will have a massage treatment of about 20 minutes. When treating small children and infants, we will do more spreading than massage – for about 10 minutes in infants and a quarter-hour in two-year-old children, and the movements will be extremely light and gentle, since in the treatment of tots, the aim of the massage is not massage for its own sake, but mainly the penetration of the oils.

Absorption of the oil during massage

The absorption of the oil into the skin and from the skin into the body depends specifically on the skin and physical build of the person who is being treated. There are people into whose skin and body the oil penetrates more easily and quickly, and others whose skin and physical build cause the oil to penetrate slowly into their body. In a healthy person, the absorption of the oils into the skin and the body is fast and easy. In a sick and injured person, and in the case of congested skin, the absorption is liable to be slower. When treating a very thin person, we must take into account that the absorption will be very rapid, and so he can sometimes be considered a child from the point of view of dosage (it depends on the degree of thinness). When treating an obese person, the absorption is likely to be slower, in accordance with the degree of obesity. When treating a very obese child, the duration of the treatment can be greatly increased.

In cases in which the client suffers from greasy or sweaty skin, a process of excretion and expelling from the body occurs, slowing down the process of penetration. For this reason, the absorption is likely to be slower.

Other points that we have to remember when giving massage treatments are that we do not give a bath treatment after a massage treatment (but it is a good idea to use an oil burner containing a pure essence of the same essential oils we used in the massage). When a client is in a state of low vitality (due to illness, old age, etc.), the blend must be further diluted by adding more carrier oil, and it is advisable to substitute oils every now and then – after two to three months of treatment with certain essential oils, according to the client's needs.

Preparing for the massage

Because the treatment with essential oils is somewhat intimate, it is important to induce a good and calm feeling in the client during the course of the treatment. The atmosphere in the room where the treatment is administered is likely to have a significant effect on the client's degree of calmness, and the calmer and more comfortable the client is, the more effective the treatment will be. To this end, we must ensure that the room is airy and smells nice. Since part of the person's body is exposed during the massage (the part that is not being massaged must be covered with a sheet or a towel; do not leave it exposed), it is important that the temperature in the room be pleasant. Cold can sabotage the massage work, since it may make the client feel uncomfortable, make it difficult for him to relax, and worst of all, contract his muscles, which can significantly jeopardize the success of the treatment. Thus, it is important to ask the client if the temperature in the room is pleasant for him, and, if necessary, to turn on the heating. (In the winter, it is important to heat the room prior to the treatment!) The lighting in the room must be dim and soothing so that the light does not disturb the client and he can doze off during the massage, if he so wishes. The addition of calm, soothing music can be wonderful during the treatment, and it is sometimes of great importance when treating people who are afraid of being touched. Whatever the case may be, it is important to ask the client if he wants to hear music, and if the type of music and the volume suit him.

The massage should be administered on a suitable bed – for both client and practitioner – a bed that affords good access to all the massage areas and does not "break" the practitioner's back. A standard treatment table is ideal for this purpose. It is no less important to make sure that the bed linen is clean and pleasant. It is preferable to use disposable sheets, since the carrier oils are likely to stain the sheet. It is very important to explain to the client that he must come to the treatment after showering, without perfumes and body lotions (this point is extremely important), and under no circumstances must he come to the treatment after a heavy meal. (Nor must he be hungry. A light meal an hour or two before the massage is recommended). In addition, it is important to remind the client to use the bathroom before the massage so that he will not feel the need during the course of the treatment. (The treatment itself stimulates evacuation, so that if someone does not relieve himself beforehand, he may feel the urge to do so during the treatment, and this will interrupt the flow!) For the sake of the client's total relaxation, it is advisable not to converse with him during the treatment. If he experiences a reaction of talkativeness, it is possible to take a short break, to rest awhile, and to continue the treatment. During the break, it is a good idea to let the client do breathing exercises or take deep abdominal breaths.

At the end of the treatment, the client must be allowed to lie quietly for a few minutes. He must get up slowly, and not suddenly or quickly. It is advisable to place a footstool under the bed if it is high, or a mat if it is low. In any case, contact of the client's feet with the cold floor should be avoided, and, if necessary, his socks and shoes should be handed to him to avoid this contact.

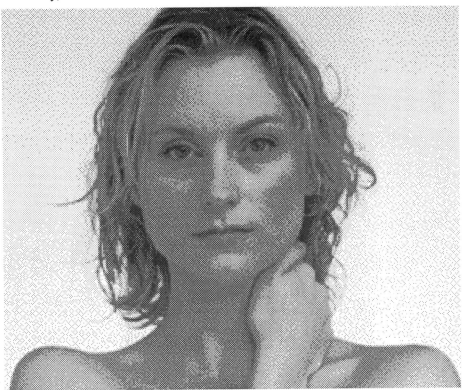

Application of essential oils

Application of the oils is performed in a similar manner to massage, except for one significant difference: the oil is spread on the skin gently, and is not massaged into it using massage movements. Application without massage is for:

treating infants, elderly people, and people with low vitality;

one of the stages of treating fractures and sprains (for more information and for an example of a combined treatment, see the section on treating sprains and sprain-like injuries);

serious cases of varicose veins;

when it is not possible to perform massage;

after surgery, when treating other areas of the body (at least two weeks after the surgery, and not on the area of the surgery or around it!);

treating bruises;

people who are not comfortable with intimate physical contact – as in massage;

cosmetic treatments, sometimes together with very gentle massage.

The application is done gently, according to the same massage dosages, but for a shorter time (since the application itself does not continue for a long time).

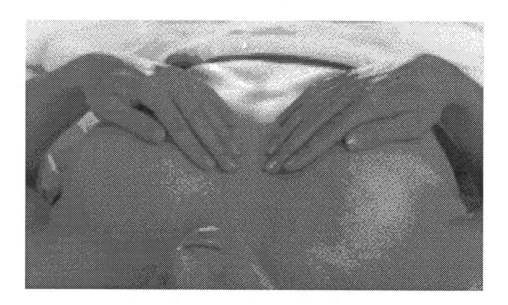

Reflexology

Reflexology is the massage of the sole of the foot – sometimes also the palm of the hand – and pressure on certain points that cause an improvement in the function of the organs that are represented by those points. Many professional reflexologists combine the use of essential oils in their reflexology treatments in order to obtain more effective results. To prepare a blend for a reflexology treatment, we apply the same rules as for preparing a blend for a massage treatment, except that the carrier oil is replaced by an identical amount of special reflexology cream. There are reflexology practitioners who do not like to administer treatment with reflexology cream, so they use a blend of carrier and essential oils, just like in a massage treatment.

Having said that, preparing a suitable blend with carrier oils is not always appropriate, especially if the foot in question has hard skin or tough calluses, since the permeability is likely to be inadequate. In that case, cream has to be used.

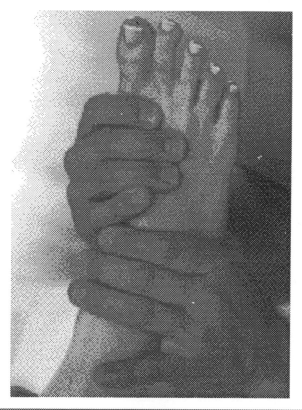

As a rule, even when a reflexology treatment is not combined with aromatherapy, it is always advisable to drip a drop of **tea tree** oil into the massage cream, since it is highly antibacterial and antiviral, and has an amazing antiseptic action. This oil protects the practitioner from eczema or fungal infections that may be present on the client's feet, and also encourages the health of the sole of the foot and protects the client himself from contracting fungal infections and eczema.

A massage must not be performed after a reflexology treatment, nor should the client take a bath with essential oils until the following day.

All the previous instructions regarding the treatment room and the client's preparations prior to treatment also pertain to reflexology treatments.

In addition, it is important to advise the client to come to the treatment with clipped toenails and a pedicure, if necessary. (In simple cases of hard skin, it is a good idea to recommend that he soak his feet in warm water for a few minutes either at home or before the treatment.)

It is also important to tell female clients to remove any nail varnish from their toenails prior to treatment.

It is a good idea to know in advance whether the client suffers from any fungal condition or eczema on his feet. In simple cases, **tea tree** oil can be mixed into the cream or massage oil. In more serious cases, the practitioner must spread a "glove cream" on his hands. This is a special cream that prevents the skin of the hands from being infected with the eczema or fungal infections on the client's feet.

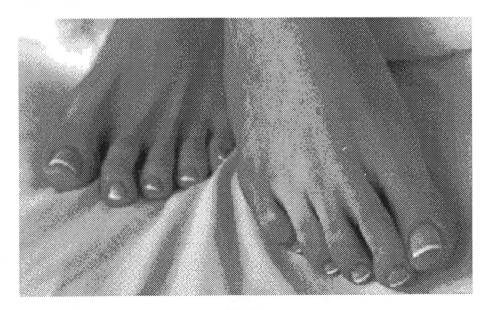

Compresses

The use of compresses is an ancient and effective way of treating many problems, and is an effective method of getting oils to penetrate the skin. Compresses are used in cases in which massage or application of the oils is not suitable, such as chills, inflammations, fractures, and sprains. The treatment with essential oils using compresses is very effective for treating pets, too (especially dogs), since the essential oils are diluted in water, instead of in oil, and do not dirty the fur or make it sticky. With dogs, treatment with compresses containing essential oils is used mainly against parasites such as fleas, for alleviating various inflammations, and for relieving pains after injuries and accidents (not on open wounds, of course). The essential oil significantly improves the natural coping mechanisms of the animal's body and helps it heal relatively quickly. This treatment must be administered gently and patiently, without frightening the animal. The dosage is determined according to the weight of the animal (small dogs – like infants; medium dogs – like children; and big dogs – like big children; a dog that weighs over 40 kilos can be given the same treatment as a human adult.) Although this book deals with aromatherapy for human beings, it is important to know about the possibility of treating household pets, since it produces excellent results. Of course, in serious animal diseases, the treatment must go hand-in-hand with proper veterinary care.

In aromatherapy using compresses, two types of compresses are generally used: hot compresses, which are mainly used in the treatment of chronic conditions that have been going on for a long time; and cold compresses, which are generally used for the treatment of acute conditions. In conditions that do not belong to either of these categories, or if it is difficult to decide which kind of compress to use, it is advisable to use a lukewarm compress, tending to cold or hot, depending on the circumstances.

Preparing the compress: In order to prepare a "whole" quantity for treating an adult, 2-3 drops of pure essential oil (with no carrier oil) must be mixed with half a liter of water. Soak cotton or a piece of cotton fabric in the water and place it on the area for 12-15 minutes.

When treating big children, mix 1-2 drops of the blend of essential oils with half a liter of water and soak cotton or a piece of cotton fabric in the water and place it on the area for about 10 minutes.

When treating small children, mix just 1 drop of essential oil or of a blend of essential oils with half a liter of water and soak cotton or a piece of cotton fabric in the water and place it on the area for 3-6 minutes.

Compresses can be applied up to three times a day, but if a massage has been given the same day, the compress should be applied only once.

Baths

Treatment using essential oils in a bath is a wonderful way of treating skin problems, of improving the appearance and vitality of the skin, of relieving pains, of lowering fever (but not when the client's condition requires medical intervention), of relaxing physically and mentally, and of treating a wide variety of emotional problems. Soaking in a bath with essential oils engenders a relaxing and enjoyable feeling. For this reason, it is also recommended for people who do not suffer from any particular problem, but simply want to relax, get rid of stress, and nurture their skin.

> **Quantities and duration of a treatment with a big bath:**
> When treating an adult, 7-8 drops of essential oils are added to the bathwater. The person must remain in the water for between 15 and 20 minutes.
> When treating big children, 4-5 drops of essential oil are added to the water, and the child must remain in the water for 10 minutes.
> When treating small children, 2-3 drops of essential oil are added to the water, and the child must remain in the water for 5-7 minutes, according to the child's age and physical condition.

There are a number of rules pertaining to treatment using essential oils in a bath: actual washing (with soap, etc.) must be done before the aromatic bath, since this bath is not followed by soaping and rinsing. Its aim is to let the oils mixed into the bathwater, remain on the skin and not reduce their action by washing them off. It is not advisable to dry oneself vigorously, but simply to wrap oneself up in a towel and go and rest. Resting after a bath containing essential oils is very important for the continued action of the oils on the body, so it is a good idea to have the bath before going to bed. In any case, it is essential to rest for at least an hour after the bath.

There are several types of baths used in aromatherapy. The first is the "big bath," which is recommended for enjoyment, freshening up, relaxation, and for any problem that requires the treatment of a large area of skin or of the entire body. In cases of a high fever, the bath should be taken in cold water.

The counter-indications for a bath include cases of high or unstable blood pressure, states of low vitality, heart diseases, post-coronary conditions, post-surgical conditions, and cases in which the person has a pacemaker. Baths should not be used after cerebral hemorrhages, either. This treatment can be administered to the elderly (only those with medium to high vitality) and children (only when it is supervised).

When treating infants, 1-2 drops of essential oil mixed with the same quantity of carrier oil are added to the water (the oils are mixed prior to the bath, and the prepared blend of essential and carrier oils is dripped into the bath), and the infant must remain in the water for up to 10 minutes.

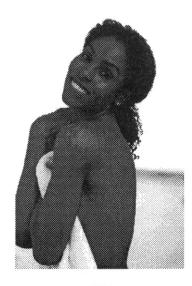

Frequency of the treatments

During the first week, treatment with a big bath can be administered daily. During the second week, it can be administered every second day. During the third and subsequent weeks, the frequency is reduced to twice a week for several weeks. When the treatment is administered over a long period of time, only one bath a week should be taken.

It is advisable to work with the same blend for two or three months, and then take a break of about a month, and substitute oils.

One of the problems posed by treatment with essential oils in the bath is the fact that the oil that is dripped into the water does not dissolve, but rather floats on the surface of the water, and its undiluted state can irritate the skin. Moreover, because of this property, it is not evenly distributed throughout the volume of the water. There are several methods of overcoming this limitation:

The essential oil can be mixed with salt (cooking salt, sea salt, bath salts, or Dead Sea salts) as follows: for every heaped tablespoon of salt, drip five drops of essential oil. In order to use a greater number of drops of essential oil (as you remember, up to seven or eight drops for an adult), it is advisable to use two tablespoons of salt. Dissolve the salt containing the drops of oil in a cup of lukewarm water, and pour it gently into the bathwater. Whatever the case may be, do not drip the oils into the empty bathtub first and then add the water – always drip them into an bathtub that is already filled with water.

Another simpler way is to drip the oil into a tablespoon of shampoo, liquid soap or liquid bubble bath, the proportion being one or two drops of oil to every tablespoon of the above liquids. When using this method, the blend of the oil with the shampoo or liquid soap can be added while the bath is filling in order to create a fragrant bubble bath.

Another method, which also contributes to skin nutrition, is to add the blend of essential oils to a tablespoon of honey. The proportion is one tablespoon of honey to one or two drops of essential oil. Here, too, it is preferable to add the honey and oil blend to the bath while it is filling (as opposed to the regular method in which the oils are dripped only after the bathtub is full, and are mixed into the bathwater by hand). Besides its effectiveness in distributing the essential oils throughout the bathwater, this method also contributes to skin nutrition, and is therefore highly recommended for a bath in order to improve the appearance of the skin. Of course, people who are allergic to honey must not use this method.

Sitz bath

Another kind of bath that is used for aromatherapy treatments is the sitz bath. In order to take a sitz bath, fill a large basin or bowl with water, mix essential oils into the water, and sit in the basin. This treatment is recommended for hemorrhoids, vaginal infections and yeast infections, and after giving birth.

Drip 4-5 drops of a blend of essential oils into a large basin or bowl containing water, and sit in the basin for 10-15 minutes. This treatment is suitable for adults only. In a therapeutic situation, this treatment can be administered daily for two weeks, followed by a two-week break for observing the developments. If there is still a need, the treatment can be resumed after the break. If there is an improvement, the bath should be taken on alternate days.

Foot bath

A foot bath is another way of getting essential oils to penetrate the skin via a bath. Widely used in aromatherapy, it is highly recommended for tired feet, fungal infections, eczema, and so on, as well as for softening hard skin prior to a reflexology treatment or a pedicure. In this treatment, too, fill a basin with lukewarm water, and drip 4-5 drops of essential oil into it. Let the feet soak for 10-15 minutes, then gently dry them and leave them free and airing for at least an hour. This treatment is suitable for adults only. As with a sitz bath treatment, this treatment can also be administered daily for the first two weeks, but only if the state of the feet is really serious (hard skin that makes it difficult to walk, eczema or fungal infections that are spreading, and so on). In less serious conditions, the treatment is administered on alternate days, or twice a week. In a therapeutic situation, in which the feet are treated in a foot bath on a daily basis, a one- to two-week break should be taken after two weeks in order to reevaluate the situation and determine the extent of improvement. The treatment is resumed after the break in accordance with the diagnosis, but only about three times a week.

An example of a combined treatment consisting of compresses, baths, application, and massage is in the treatment of light fractures (after the plaster cast has been removed) and sprains: During the first stage, when the pain is intense or some time after the cast has been removed, use essential oils in the form of compresses and cold local baths, or "big" lukewarm baths.

During the second stage, use gentle application in order to assist healing and assuage the pain.

During the third stage, it is possible to move on to massage, according to the state of the injured person.

Oil burner

The oil burner is one of the most common methods of using essential oils. In the sections dealing with the mental aspects that are treated with aromatherapy, you can see the beneficial action of the oils on the body and mind via inhalation of the oil vapors. The simple preparation of the oil burner for treatment makes it convenient and effective in every situation.

The oil burner is generally made of clay. Its upper part contains a saucer that can either be separate from or attached to the rest of the burner, in which water (preferably mineral water) is placed. Essential oil is dripped into the water. In the lower part of the burner, there is an opening in which a small candle is placed (the candle that is used in a burner is small, low, round, and in an aluminum container, thus preventing the burner from being spattered with melted wax). Sometimes these candles are called "tea candles," and they are available in almost every grocery store. When the candle is lit, it warms the saucer and the water in it. Within a few minutes, the steam from the oil rises and permeates the room.

The amount of oil used in the burner is 3-12 drops of the blend (according to the size of the room in which the burner is placed) in the saucer of water on the burner – extremely simple! Its use is not limited – it can be used even four or five times a day (although this should not be overdone, either).

The uses of a burner are numerous. In principle, we use a burner for any treatment in which we are also treating the mental aspect of the client – for alleviating tension and stress, nervousness, bad moods, fatigue, exhaustion, memory problems, and problems with studying for exams, for increasing alertness, concentration, and sexual arousal, for cleansing the room of non-positive energies or unpleasant odors, and many more.

The burner can also be used for treating respiratory diseases. We might use inhalation for the treatment of a specific problem in the respiratory system, but since this method cannot be used many times a day, it is advisable to drip some of the aromatic blend into the burner in order to obtain better results from the treatment. Moreover, the use of an oil burner is significant when one of the family has a bacterial or viral disease. In such cases, it is important to place a blend of suitable antiviral or antibacterial oils in the burner in order to disinfect the air in the house and prevent it from becoming contaminated.

The use of a burner containing a suitable blend of essential oils can also be wonderful for social events (for instance, when you choose uplifting oils such as **bergamot**) and for romantic encounters (as we shall see in the section on sexual arousal). There are people who are in the habit of placing a burner containing oils that enhance alertness and concentration, or soothing oils that create a pleasant atmosphere, in their workplace. In kindergartens, too, putting a burner *in a place that is inaccessible to the children* contributes greatly to a calm, comfortable atmosphere. During "epidemics" of flu, colds, and so on, it is a good idea to place a blend of appropriate antibacterial or antiviral oils in the burner.

Dripping 2-3 drops of **lavender** oil is suitable for almost everyone, and the smell of the **lavender** that permeates the room creates a calm, tranquil, and pleasant mood along with a pleasing odor. **Lavender** oil is recommended, since it treats an extremely broad range of problems, and also fortifies the immune system. Moreover, there is hardly anyone who does not benefit from the fragrant **lavender** vapors in the room.

When using an oil burner, you must watch out for several "heavier" essential oils that sink rather than float on the surface of the water. When using **clove**, **benzoin** or **sandalwood** oil, for instance, it is advisable to drip the oil onto the side of the saucer, above the waterline, in order to prevent it from sinking to the bottom of the saucer.

A very important point regarding the use of an oil burner: When we purchase a burner, under no circumstances must either burner or saucer be made of metal. While burners of this type are indeed sold in nature and New Age stores, the metal reacts with the aromatic blend, and this has unhealthy effects.

It is extremely important to clean the burner with hot water and detergent after use, and sometimes it is advisable to soak it for a while in hot water and scrub its saucer with half a lemon in order to get rid of the stains caused by the recently-used oils. This problem is common mainly in clay burners that are glazed, after the candle has burned for a long time, and also after the water has almost completely evaporated. In these cases, an odoriferous accumulation of essential oil residues is formed, and this can interfere with the action of the new blend that is placed in the oil burner.

It is important to mention that nowadays, various synthetic blends sold in stores are described as "For use in oil burners." These blends are in no way suitable for treatment, even though some of them may be labeled "Oil for meditation," "Erotic oil," etc. When the oil is synthetic or mixed with synthetic components, these claims are generally nonsense, since the oils have absolutely no effect other than giving the room a pleasant fragrance. Experienced practitioners will immediately distinguish the presence of synthetic components in an essential oil. Whoever cannot distinguish them should buy only from a reputed essential oil supplier.

Another problem caused by synthetic blends is that they leave such a strong smell in the saucer of the burner that it is sometimes difficult to get rid of it. Therefore it is highly recommended to avoid using a burner in which these spurious blends have been dripped for therapeutic purposes.

A burner can and should be used in conjunction with the other treatments such as massage, baths, and so on, and it is always advisable for the blend of oils in the burner (a pure blend, without carrier oil) to be identical to or contain some of the oils that were used in the other treatments. In any event, it is not a good idea to add other oils to the burner in excess of the four (maximum) that were used in the other treatments. In the case of three or less essential oils, it is possible to add one more essential oil to the burner, if our desired goal is not characterized by the oils we chose for the treatment.

Inhalation

Inhalation is used mainly for treating problems of the respiratory system. It helps open the respiratory passages, treat viral flu and a broad range of viral diseases, and humidify the air.

For inhalation, we can prepare an "instrument" using good, old-fashioned methods: a bowl of about a liter of hot but not boiling water that emits steam, and 4-5 drops of a blend of essential oils dripped into it. As the treatment progresses, another drop or two can be added, as needed. The person's head is covered with a towel and bent over the bowl so that the steam is trapped and directed toward his face and respiratory organs, and he inhales the steam for a few minutes. In cases of colds, flu, chills, and so on, it is possible to administer this treatment daily, and sometimes once in the morning and once in the evening (before going to sleep), in order to attain significant relief. A steam appliance can be used in the same way. Four drops are dripped into the appliance, or into a special opening in the appliance, and the person inhales for a few minutes. Today, it is also possible to purchase inhalation appliances that are especially suitable for the inhalation of essential oils, and they are very effective. (In addition, it is possible to administer a *cleansing facial treatment*, which moisturizes and softens the skin, by preparing a suitable cosmetic blend, and holding the face over the bowl containing hot water.)

Another method of inhaling steam that contains essential oil, which is mainly effective for treating infants, small children, and people who are unable to use inhalation (there are many people who do not feel comfortable with the steam and heat that rise from the bowl), is dripping a drop or two of the essential oil or

Caution! Counter-indications for the use of inhalation: asthma sufferers. Before recommending the use of inhalation to someone, we first find out whether he suffers from asthma. Even if he reports a respite of several months since his last attack, don't be tempted and don't try it! The steam can irritate the respiratory system of asthma sufferers and bring on an asthma attack.

blend on a handkerchief or tissue, and sniffing it; or dripping one drop of suitable essential oil on the pillow (for an adult, two or three drops can be used; for children and infants – one drop). This method is wonderful for treating infants with colds.

It is also possible to drip one drop of calming oil that is suitable for use with infants – **neroli**, **chamomile**, **lavender**, **niaouli**, or **frankincense**, for instance – on the pillow, in order to calm the infant down or facilitate sleep.

Vaginal douches

Vaginal douches are used to clean the vagina when there are yeast and other infections, vaginal candida, and so on. The douche is also good after menstruation and after intercourse. There are women who suffer from recurrent urinary tract infections when they have intercourse, probably because of bacteria that reside in her partner, but do not bother him.

Generally, these urinary tract infections occur after the first few instances of intercourse, when the women is "learning to know" the bacteria. This condition is called "Honeymoon cystitis," and, in such cases, it is extremely important to use a douche after sex.

The vaginal douche is performed using a douche-bag, an appliance that is similar in shape to a rubber enema, except smaller. (A new rubber enema will serve the purpose well.) The plastic nozzle must be washed very well before use, then the rubber bag is filled with a blend of essential oils and water, the nozzle is inserted into the vagina, and the douche-bag is squeezed so that water sprays into the vaginal passage.

To prepare the douche liquid, take a cup of lukewarm water, add a teaspoon of salt, plus 2-3 drops of the aromatic blend. Instead of salt, two tablespoons of vinegar can be added to the water.

Another way of preparing the douche liquid is by boiling laurel leaves, chamomile, or sage. Wait until the liquid has cooled to lukewarm, and then essential oils can be dripped into a cup of the liquid. Pour the water or the liquid mixed with the aromatic blend into the rubber douche-bag (a small funnel can be used for this).

During the first days of the treatment of yeast or other vaginal infections, it is advisable to perform between two and three douches a day, and one douche a day for two more days after that.

An example of a blend for treating yeast infections contains one drop of **lavender** oil, one drop of **myrrh** oil, and one drop of **tea tree** oil.

An example of a blend for treating a vaginal infection contains one drop of **chamomile** oil, one drop of **bergamot** oil, and one drop of **eucalyptus** oil.

In any case, it is very advisable not to perform protracted or daily treatments with a douche-bag over any length of time. The vagina contains essential fluids and lubricants, and the frequent use of a douche can dry them up. For this reason, it should only be used when necessary.

An additional, perhaps "home" remedy for treating yeast and other vaginal infections is a tampon coated with carrier oil. Drip up to two drops of a suitable aromatic blend on the tampon. Spread the blend well over the tampon. Insert the tampon, and remove it after an hour or two.

Strange as this may sound, applying bio yogurt (yogurt that contains "friendly" bacteria) to the tampon and using it as described above (without the essential oils) obtains impressive results in the treatment of the symptoms of urinary tract infections. Tampons should not be used more than twice a day, and can be used alternately with a vaginal douche – one remedy on one day, and another on the next day – but not both remedies on the same day.

As we said before, these are treatments for vaginal "emergencies" only, when there is a painful burning sensation. *It is important to be examined by a physician*, especially in cases of recurrent urinary tract infections (remember that these recurrent infections can damage the kidneys), and in cases of candida, it is imperative to consult a suitable practitioner, naturopath, a healer with therapeutic plants or a dietician. (Many physicians do not have the correct and suitable treatment for candida, other than antibiotics, which themselves are one of the main causes of the growth of candida!) The candida infection has many different symptoms, and affects many bodily systems. For this reason, it must under no circumstances be neglected. Candida causes many symptoms in the various bodily systems. Treating it may well make these symptoms (which do not seem to be in the least linked to the candida itself, but actually stem from it) vanish, as if by magic. This results in a significant change in the person's state of health.

Mouthwashes

Mouthwashes are used in cases of oral infections and inflammations, gum infections, throat infections, inflamed mouth ulcers, abscesses (stemming from a lack of vitamins and a weak immune system), after tooth extractions, and in cases of halitosis originating in either the mouth or in the digestive system.

For treating oral infections, the following essential oils are recommended: **chamomile, lavender,** and **bergamot,** and for treatment following tooth extractions, it is advisable to gargle with one or two of the following oils: **lavender, geranium, cypress,** and **lemon. Lemon** and **cypress** oils are astringent oils – that is, they shrink blood vessels – and are therefore effective in stopping bleeding.

The liquid for gargling and rinsing the mouth is prepared from a glass of lukewarm water, a cup of herb tea, or a cup of water in which laurel leaves have been boiled. Two or three drops of essential oils are dripped into the liquid. The mouth is rinsed well with the mixture, which is then gargled and spit out, two or three times a day. The disinfectant effect can be enhanced by adding a bit of squeezed lemon juice or a half-teaspoon of salt to the gargling liquid.

It must be remembered that using mouthwashes for gum infections, halitosis as a result of digestive tract or teeth problems, abscesses, and sore throats, is symptomatic treatment only – it relieves the symptoms of the diseases, but does not cure it. It is therefore important to combine the mouthwashes with a suitable and comprehensive plan of treatment, and, of course, when necessary, to clarify the reasons for halitosis, and treat the digestive tract or visit the dentist accordingly.

4

Warnings

Among the essential oils, there are various oils that are not suitable for the treatment of children and infants, pregnant women, or epileptics. There are phototoxic oils – that is, skin that has been treated with these oils must not be exposed to sunlight for 12 hours following treatment; there are oils that may irritate sensitive skin (therefore, we must do a patch test – put a drop on the client's skin, then wait for 15 minutes to see that there is no irritation), and other negative side effects. Aromatherapy that is performed by meticulously observing the rules for treatment and the use of suitable oils is not in the least dangerous. However, for beginner practitioners (even experienced practitioners can forget) and for people who do not have professional training in aromatherapy, it is important to check every oil that has been selected for the blend against the following list of all the oils whose used is limited. The list is alphabetical.

Achillea – a phototoxic oil that must not be exposed to sunlight for 12 hours following treatment.

Angelica – a phototoxic oil that must not be exposed to sunlight for 12 hours following treatment. It must not be used during pregnancy.

Anise – must not be used during pregnancy. It has a high level of toxicity. It should be used by experienced, professional practitioners only.

Basil – must not be used during pregnancy.

Bergamot – a phototoxic oil that must not be exposed to sunlight for 12 hours following treatment. It is possible to use this oil when it is bergapten-free, since it is safer and can be exposed to sunlight after use, but its therapeutic properties may be affected.

Birch – has a high level of toxicity. It should be used by experienced, professional practitioners only.

Black pepper – must not be used during pregnancy. It must not be used on the face, since it is a very potent oil.

Cajeput – the client's skin must be tested with a drop of the oil 15 minutes before treatment in case it irritates sensitive skin.

Camphor – an oil that penetrates deeply into the cells, and must not be used for a long period of time. It has a high level of toxicity. It must not be used by people who suffer from asthma. It must not be used during pregnancy. Avoid using it in a whole-body massage. *As a rule, it should not be used at all*.

Caraway – the client's skin must be tested with a drop of the oil 15 minutes before treatment in case it irritates sensitive skin. It must not be used during pregnancy.

Cardamon – the client's skin must be tested with a drop of the oil 15 minutes before treatment in case it irritates sensitive skin.

Cedarwood – must not be used during pregnancy.

Cinnamon – has a high level of toxicity. It must not be used to treat infants and tots. It must not be used during pregnancy. Avoid using it on the face.

Clary sage – must not be used during pregnancy. Do not drive after using it. Do not drink alcohol before or after using it as it might cause unpleasant sensations and nightmares. It must not be used by women who suffer from mastitis, or by women who do not wish to increase the level of estrogen in their bodies. Having said that, **clary sage** oil is much safer for use than medicinal sage.

Clove – must not be used during pregnancy. It must not be used to treat infants and tots. Always use small amounts to avoid skin irritations.

Coriander – only a tiny amount must be used when used on the face, since it may irritate the skin.

Dill – must not be used to treat infants and tots or during pregnancy.

Eucalyptus – must not be used to treat infants and tots – in fact, its use on children in general should be avoided (**niaouli** or **myrtle** can be used instead).

Fennel – must not be used to treat infants and children up to age six. A large quantity may cause an epileptic seizure. It is not recommended for use when the estrogen level is high or when there is excessive estrogen in the body. It must not be used during pregnancy. It must not be used to treat epileptics.

Galbanum – the client's skin must be tested with a drop of the oil 15 minutes before treatment in case it irritates sensitive skin. It must not be used during pregnancy.

Garlic – the client's skin must be tested with a drop of slightly diluted oil 15 minutes before treatment in case it irritates sensitive skin. It must not be used by nursing mothers.

Extra precautions must be taken when used on the skin, since the oil is very powerful and can cause a burn.

Geranium – the client's skin must be tested with a drop of the oil 15 minutes before treatment in case it irritates sensitive skin.

Ginger – must not be used to treat infants and tots. It must be used in a highly diluted form in order to avoid skin irritations.

Grapefruit – a phototoxic oil that must not be exposed to sunlight for 12 hours following treatment.

Hyssop – has a high level of toxicity. It must not be used by pregnant women, by epileptics, by children, or by people with a high fever. *It should be used by experienced, professional practitioners only.*

Juniper – must not be used during pregnancy.

Laurel – must not be used during pregnancy.

Lemon – a phototoxic oil that must not be exposed to sunlight for 12 hours following treatment. It should not be used during the summer. The client's skin must be tested with a drop of the oil 15 minutes before treatment in case it irritates sensitive skin.

Lemongrass – must not be used to treat infants and tots. The client's skin must be tested with a drop of the oil 15 minutes before treatment in case it irritates sensitive skin. It should be used in a highly diluted form and in small quantities.

Lime – a phototoxic oil that must not be exposed to sunlight for 12 hours following treatment.

Louisa – must not be exposed to sunlight for 12 hours following treatment. It should not be used during the summer.

Mandarin – a phototoxic oil that must not be exposed to sunlight for 12 hours following treatment.

Marjoram – must not be used to treat infants or during pregnancy. It should not be used prior to driving. The client's skin must be tested with a drop of the oil 15 minutes before treatment in case it irritates sensitive skin. It should be used in a highly diluted form. No more than four drops should be used in the bath.

Melissa – must not be used during pregnancy.

Myrrh – must not be used to treat infants or during pregnancy.

Neroli – a phototoxic oil that must not be exposed to sunlight for 12 hours following treatment.

Nutmeg – must not be used during pregnancy. The client's skin must be tested with a drop of the oil 15 minutes before treatment in case it irritates sensitive skin. Do not use for long periods of time.

Orange – a phototoxic oil that must not be exposed to sunlight for 12 hours following treatment.

Parsley – must not be used during pregnancy. Always use in small quantities.

Peppermint – a large quantity prior to sleeping may induce nightmares. As a rule, it should not be used before sleep, since it is stimulating and can prevent the person from falling asleep. This oil must not be used in a whole-body massage. It may cause a sensation of extreme cold. For this reason, it should not be the only oil used in a bath, but should be combined with other oils. It must not be used during pregnancy, nor must it be used to treat infants and tots.

Red thyme – must not be used to treat infants and tots or pregnant women. It must not be used by people who suffer from hypertension. It must be used in very small quantities to avoid skin irritations.

Rosemary – must not be used during pregnancy. It raises blood pressure. It must not be used by people who suffer from unstable hypertension. For treating people with balanced or borderline high blood pressure, add this oil to a blend of oils that lowers blood pressure. It must not be used to treat epileptics.

Sage (medicinal) – must not be used to treat infants, pregnant women, or epileptics. In large quantities, it can cause an epileptic seizure, central nervous system disorders, and powerful contractions of the smooth muscles. It must not be used by people who suffer from hypertension. As a rule, it should be used by experienced, professional practitioners only.

Spearmint – must not be used during pregnancy.

Sweet thyme – must not be used during pregnancy. However, it is safer for use than red thyme.

Wintergreen – has a high level of toxicity. *It should be used by experienced, professional practitioners only.*

Yarrow – decreases the skin's protection against the sun, and should not be used during the summer for long periods. It must not be exposed to sunlight for 12 hours following treatment.

Ylang-ylang – can cause headaches when used in large quantities.

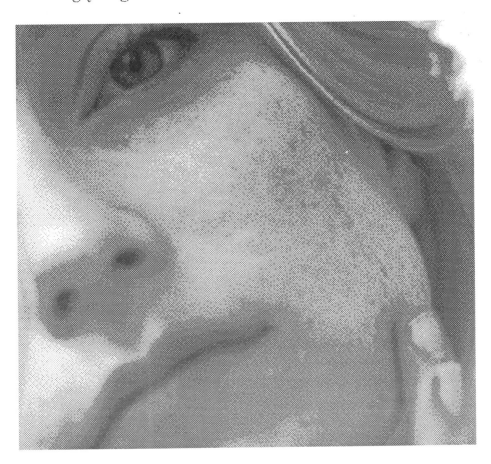

5

Aromatherapy Treatments

Halitosis

My neighbor, Dana, has suffered from inflamed gums for a long time. Her condition is being treated by her dentist, and the treatment will gradually help cure it, but in the meantime, she suffers from a very common and extremely annoying problem – halitosis.

In most cases, halitosis is not a problem on its own, but rather a secondary symptom of a more basic problem. When we treat halitosis, it is very important to examine its primary cause. This can be various digestive problems, respiratory infections, gum or tooth ailments, disorders in the digestive system, or, in many cases, defective oral hygiene. The latter means that if one does not brush one's teeth properly, bits of food, especially meat, get stuck between the teeth, begin to decay, and cause bad breath.

Sometimes, the client is meticulous about brushing his teeth properly, but because his teeth are exceptionally close together, tiny bits of food get stuck between them. In this case, the regular (and careful) use of dental floss is recommended in order to get rid of the bits of food that are not removed by regular brushing.

Even for the sake of symptomatic treatment (which does not treat the cause itself, but just the symptoms of bad breath), you must get to the root of the problem and treat it. I suggested the following treatment to Dana:

Each morning, and every time she felt that her breath was not fresh, she should drip one drop each of the essential oils of **peppermint** and **lemon** into a glass of lukewarm water. She should then gargle with the mixture a few times, *taking care not to swallow it* (for this reason, only a small amount must be gargled each time).

The **peppermint** and **lemon** mixture would freshen her breath and mouth. **Peppermint** oil would impart a fresh and pleasant odor to her mouth, and **lemon** oil, besides its compatibility from the point of view of smell, also has an extremely powerful antiseptic and disinfectant effect and destroys yeast and viruses. It could therefore help treat Dana's inflamed gums.

Dana tried gargling with the mixture a few times. She began to feel an improvement in the odor of her breath. This lasted for a few hours, and in order to safeguard herself from unpleasantness at work, she prepared a 10 cc bottle of equal quantities of **peppermint** and **lemon** oils from which she would prepare her gargling mixture. She gargled several times a day – at work, too.

It must be remembered that children under 10 must not be allowed to gargle with the mixture. From age 10 to 14, the gargling process should be supervised in order to make sure that the child is only gargling small amounts and is not swallowing them. While it is not dangerous to swallow a small amount of oil diluted in a relatively large amount of water (some aromatherapy methods advocate taking the oils orally, but they are not widespread), swallowing is not at all pleasant, and may cause a burning sensation in the throat, as well as coughing and dizziness. The feeling is similar to the one that occurs when people swallow mouthwash, and anyone who has experienced this will know that it is not pleasant. Again, while it is not dangerous, it is not fun either!

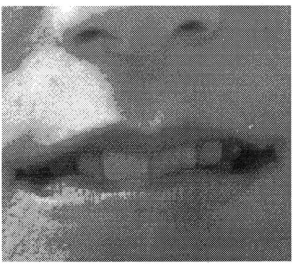

Headaches

One day, my friend Jason asked me to help him get rid of a bad headache that was bothering him. Jason owned a photographic equipment store, and his head was aching after a long day of work in which he had dealt with various irritating things. To make things worse, he was suffering terribly from the noise caused by the road repairs that were being carried out near his store by City Hall – an ear-splitting noise that stopped every once in a while and then resumed more fiercely than ever. Jason had gone home agitated, with an annoying headache that he had tried to relieve by sitting in front of the TV with a cup of tea. However, he soon realized that the pain had not disappeared at all. Of course, he could have taken a pill to relieve the headache, and this might have helped, but he objects on principle to taking medications without a really good reason for doing so. (He's right. There are many cases that do not justify the ingestion of harmful chemical substances, and it is a shame to become accustomed to using pills, since they are not good for the body.) He was prepared to wait for several hours for the pain to disappear, but on second thoughts, decided to try aromatherapy – perhaps it would get rid of the headache that was bothering him.

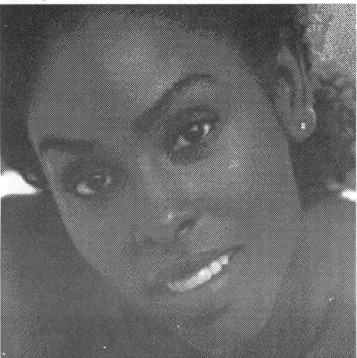

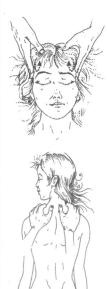

Headaches can be brought on by a very wide range of causes. When a headache stems from agitation, fatigue, nasal congestion, and so on, aromatherapy may be of great help in alleviating the pain. When a headache is especially bad or protracted, or is the result of a blow, it is essential to be examined and treated by a physician. In order to treat headaches that are caused by sinusitis, colds, fatigue and migraine, it is advisable to administer the treatment described in this book (in the sections dealing with these problems).

In order to treat routine headaches, it is advisable to perform a local massage on the shoulders, the neck, the temples, and gently around the eyes. For Jason, I prepared a mixture of one tablespoon of **almond** carrier oil and one drop of **chamomile** essential oil. It is also possible to use one drop of **lavender** essential oil. Moreover, I suggested that he choose two or more of the following essential oils for use in an oil burner: **chamomile**, **lavender**, **eucalyptus**, **lemon**, or **peppermint**. We would place a total of 12 drops of the oils he chose in the burner. After smelling the oils, he asked me to light a burner containing the following oils: **lavender**, **chamomile**, and **peppermint**.

Jason sat in my apartment for about an hour and a half, during which time I performed a gentle massage that began on his forehead, went down to his temples in gentle circular movements, continued to his eyebrows and carefully around his eyes, then to his cheekbones, and lastly down to his neck and the nape.

A wonderful way of treating the nape of the neck is as follows: The person lies down, and you stand behind him. Spread the blend of oils on both your hands, gently hold the base of his neck (where it joins his shoulders), and perform gentle pulling movements toward you by drawing your hands slowly along the surface of the back of the neck and head. If the person has long hair, loosen the hair, shake it a bit, and pull it gently. You can also massage his scalp with all your fingers (if he doesn't mind his hair becoming a bit oily), using gentle shampooing movements. After a relaxing and releasing massage of the neck and scalp, move on to his shoulders, using pushing and (gentle) pinching movements of the whole palm for releasing the tense and contracted shoulder muscles.

Jason lay resting on the treatment table with the sounds of calm, quiet, slightly meditative music in the background, and the essential oil vapor filling the room. Since he was tired from the day's work, and the effect of the essential oil massage was so soothing, he dozed off for about an hour. When he awoke, he was limp and relaxed, and his headache had disappeared.

When the treatment for a headache includes massage along with an oil burner and rest in a pleasant and relaxing atmosphere, the effectiveness of the treatment increases significantly. Jason went home without a headache, feeling content and calm.

In cases in which success is not so rapid, and the headache continues even after massage, you can wait an hour and repeat the massage in order to derive greater benefit from the treatment and significant relief from the headache.

Migraines

Judy came for an aromatherapy treatment because of the severe migraines she had been suffering from for years. She was 52 years old, a psychotherapist by profession, and the mother of three grown children. She described the migraine attacks as terrible suffering that neutralized her to the point that she was unable to function for several hours – sometimes almost an entire day – and was forced to cancel her appointments.

A migraine is an extremely disturbing ailment that is common among children and young people and generally disappears after age 50. However, there are many people who suffer from it most of their lives. It is a disease with a family history, and it may be linked to genetic factors. In women, the migraine can be linked to conditions such as pregnancy and menstruation. The migraine is characterized by the onslaught of headaches that generally begin on one side of the head and then spread over the entire head. The attacks can last for anything from a few minutes to several days, and their frequency varies from person to person – between several attacks a week and a single attack every few months. During the attack, the person is in a state of tension and restlessness, suffers from nausea, vomiting, constipation or diarrhea, and is hypersensitive to light and noise. In some cases, there are various sensations that precede the attack (these sensations are called an "aura"), so the person knows that he is about to have a migraine attack. Among them are: a mood swing, tingling in the hands, sight disruptions that include flashing lights and geometric shapes in the field of vision, and sometimes weakness in half of the body. These signs appear in parallel to contractions of the cerebral blood vessels. Migraine headaches are caused by changes in the diameter of the blood vessels. In the period preceding the pain, the blood vessels contract, and during the pain, they expand.

There are certain factors that can cause a migraine attack. These include: bright lights, loud noise, certain odors, foods such as chocolate or yellow cheese, tension, and menstruation. Migraines are usually treated with medications. Since the pain is caused when the blood vessels expand, the treatment administered is medication that shrinks the blood vessels. In less severe cases, light pain relievers are used. More severe cases are treated with stronger medications, which, unfortunately, have serious side-effects and are not always effective. However, in cases where treatment with medication is effective, it can – if it is administered in time – preempt the stage in which the blood vessels expand, thereby preventing the headache.

Aromatherapy can greatly alleviate migraine pain. It is important to use the oils as soon as the feeling of migraine begins in order to prevent or diminish the attack.

I prepared a blend of the following oils for Judy: I poured 30 cc of **apricot kernel** oil into a 30-cc bottle. Since the massage is performed on the forehead and temples, I chose a mainly cosmetic oil that is pleasant to spread on the face. From the essential oils, I selected **chamomile** oil, which is soothing, anesthetizing, antispasmodic (prevents contractions), and suitable for sensitive facial skin that tends to redness, like Judy's. I dripped six drops of **chamomile** oil into the bottle, and then added six drops of **lavender** oil, which is soothing, analgesic (pain-relieving), and helps alleviate neurological pains. The third oil I chose was **peppermint** oil, which is also antispasmodic, and is known to be very effective with headaches.

I asked Judy to apply the oil to her forehead and temples the moment she felt the beginning of a migraine attack, and to massage her temples gently while taking deep, comfortable, and slow abdominal breaths.

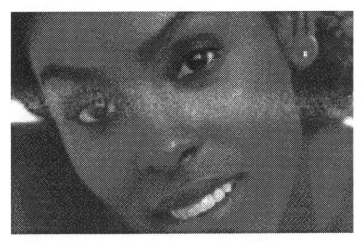
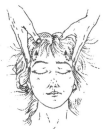

Judy found it difficult to believe that the oils would help her migraine attacks. She had tried everything, and her faith had worn thin. However, she was prepared to try anything in order to find a way to cope with her problem. She placed the bottle in one of her kitchen closets so that it would be easily available. A few days after receiving the blend, she felt the onset of an attack. It was early in the morning, and she was preparing some breakfast for herself.

Suddenly she felt a light prickling sensation in her limbs, followed immediately by a disturbing dizziness. She hurried over to the closet, grabbed the bottle of oil, sat down, and tried to calm down. She tended to become stressed out at the beginning of a migraine attack because she dreaded the terrible, all-too-familiar pain she would soon be suffering. She poured a little oil into her hands, spread it over her temples in circular movements, spread a bit on her forehead with outward stretching movements, and then resumed massaging her temples for about 15 minutes. The massage and the effect of the oils made her drowsy, so she got into bed to rest after darkening the room and closing the door to prevent light or noise from increasing her pain and discomfort.

Since she was tired, she fell asleep, waking up two hours later. To her astonishment, she only had a slight headache on the left side of her head. She was still not sure enough of herself to get up and function normally because she was afraid that the pain might intensify. However, it gradually decreased, disappearing an hour and a half later, and she could get on with her day as usual.

Since then, she uses the blend every time she feels the onset of a migraine. While she has not had total relief, and still suffers from migraines for several hours, the pain is much less severe and intense than the pain she endured in the past. Things that used to disturb her and intensify the pain during the migraine, such as movement, light, or noise, bother her much less now.

She also says that the attacks are shorter, and she needs less time to get back into full swing. Having said that, she still feels the need to rest during the migraine, and usually rests for about two hours. Sometimes she takes one pill to relieve the headache, and this, together with massaging her temples with the blend, affords her significant relief. In the past, she would take three pills for the headache, almost without getting any relief. To her joy, she has even discovered that the actual application of the oil is not only very pleasant – it actually improves the appearance of her facial skin (even though the blend was not prepared specifically for that purpose). For this reason, she sometimes spreads the blend over her face to treat the skin. Sometimes, when she is not suffering from a migraine, but is just tense or nervous, she applies the oil to her temples and experiences calmness and a decrease in tension and nervousness.

Stomach pains

There are many different reasons for stomach pains. When a client complains of stomach pains, it is very important to determine the source of the pain and, accordingly, send him for medical tests. It is important to use a process of elimination in order to find the basic cause of the pain. Later on, we will present several common problems in the digestive system that cause stomach pains, and the methods of treating them with essential oils.

It must be remembered that stomach pains, when they are out of the ordinary, inexplicable or disproportionate, or perpetual and disturbing, must be examined and treated by a physician. This is also the case when the stomach pain is accompanied by a high fever, diarrhea, headaches, and other symptoms. There can be many reasons for stomach pains, among them overeating, poor nutrition, eating too fast, consuming very spicy food, menstrual pains, constipation, muscle pains, flatulence, and so on. When a stomach pain results from one of the above causes, and it is annoying but not too severe, it can be treated with natural remedies.

A friend of mine, who is not too particular about regular meals or what he eats, calls me up every now and then to ask my advice about a slight stomach pain that occasionally disrupts his crowded schedule.

Although the pains are not especially severe or significant, he has undergone medical tests that did not reveal any pathological findings. Apparently, they are caused by incorrect eating, by foods that are not compatible with his body and state of health, or by incorrect food combinations. In parallel to preparing an aromatherapy treatment for his problem, I asked him, of course, to consult with a dietician in order to regulate his daily menu – this would cancel out possibilities of intolerance to certain foods and thus solve the problem at its root.

As a symptomatic treatment, the treatment of ordinary stomach pains with essential oils is very effective. First of all, the person with the pains is advised to drink a soothing herbal tea, such as chamomile tea, sage tea, or peppermint tea, which help relieve stomach pains. Infusions of the herbs themselves (they can be purchased in health stores) can be much more effective than the herbal teabags sold in supermarkets. The tea must be sipped slowly, and then the person should rest for a few minutes.

After the rest, a massage of the abdominal region can be performed, using a blend that contains one tablespoon of **sunflower** oil and one drop of **chamomile** oil.

The massage must not be performed with powerful or invasive movements, but rather with gentle circular and spreading movements. My friend used the blend after he had drunk a tea made from an infusion of chamomile flowers. He massaged his abdomen with gentle movements for 15 minutes, and, after a short rest lying down, he felt a great relief in his stomach pains. After a few hours, he resumed his normal activities.

It is important to remember that resuming normal activities directly after feeling relief is not advisable. The person should continue resting, or, at the very least, not resume any activity that raises the level of mental stress or tension, or that requires him to strain his body or his stomach muscles.

This blend is also suitable for stomach pains in children and infants, since it is very mild and diluted. However, when treating children and infants, we do not perform a massage, but simply spread the blend over their abdomen for a few minutes (5-10 minutes, according to the child's age), using gentle, soothing movements. Before doing so, we should give the child or infant a little chamomile tea to drink (it can be put in the baby's bottle, and given to him when it is lukewarm).

For other treatments of stomach pains resulting from specific causes, see the sections that follow.

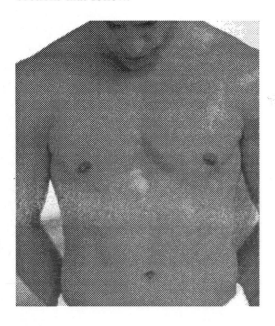
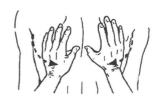

Peptic ulcer

Stomach pains may be caused by an ulcer located either in the stomach or in the duodenum. A peptic ulcer is the damage to and destruction of a very small part of the covering tissue of the stomach, the duodenum, or the esophagus. The ulcer is usually single, but there are conditions in which there are multiple ulcers. Generally, duodenal ulcers are the most common. Stomach ulcers are caused by impairment of the ability of the mucosa (the covering tissue of the stomach) to defend itself against the salicylic acid in the stomach, while duodenal ulcers are caused by excessive acidity from the stomach. There are a number of causes for the formation of ulcers, and it is important to inform the client of the causes that are in his control. One of the most common causes is the Helicobacter pylori bacterium that is found in the stomachs of 40% of the population. It lives in the stomach acids, and causes stomach ulcers in some of the people in whom it resides. As aromatherapists, our contribution to the treatment of this condition is by strengthening the immune system.

Another very common cause of ulcers is smoking. In addition, alcohol and certain medications, which are called ulcerogenic because of their action, are also known to cause ulcers. All the medications for joints and muscles that must be taken with food may also cause stomach ulcers or aggravate existing stomach ulcers, as are corticosteroids and medications for non-steroidal inflammations.

In addition, one of the common causes of ulcers is the type A personality – career-oriented, tense, and nervous people. Ulcers often occur in people of this type, and it is well-known that states of stress and tension aggravate the condition and cause stomach pains in ulcer sufferers. Aromatherapy plays a significant role in reducing stress as well.

The hereditary factor also needs to be mentioned, since certain families have a greater tendency to form ulcers, as well as the fact that the disease is more widespread among men and generally occurs during adulthood. According to estimates, the disease afflicts 10% of the population.

When diagnosing the ulcer (before the medical exam confirms the findings), we must be familiar with the symptoms that characterize the problem: the pain mainly occurs in the epigastrium (upper abdominal region) below the tip of the sternum (breastbone). If there is a flow of gastric acid from the stomach to the esophagus (a condition called gastro-esophageal reflux), the client will complain of pains and/or heartburn behind the sternum. If complications in the ulcer occur, and it penetrates in the direction of the pancreas, the pain may radiate to the back. Clients tend to describe the pain as burning, pressing, irksome, cutting, cramping, a feeling of hunger – or conversely, a feeling of fullness in the stomach and hiccups – in short, a pain that can cause nausea and vomiting. The pain lasts for relatively short lengths of time, but occurs for periods of several weeks at a time, alternating with periods of respite. In general, the pain is more severe when there is an increased secretion of acid and there is no food in the stomach to counteract the acid (by diluting it): several hours after eating and at night. Antacid medications relieve the pain, so does eating and drinking non-acidic food and liquid. Generally, food intensifies the pain of the stomach ulcer and relieves the pain of the duodenal ulcer.

There are clients who complain of nausea, a lack of appetite, or vomiting. In contrast, there are those for whom there is no clear clinical picture of an ulcer, and they show up at the physician's consulting room for the first time with complications. The complications resulting from an untreated stomach ulcer can be very dangerous. Therefore, it is extremely important to diagnose the disease and treat it at an early stage. Among the common complications are: the strangulation of the stomach or the duodenum and the emptying of the stomach contents into the abdominal cavity; the downward growth of the ulcer and damage to a large blood vessel, resulting in hemorrhaging in the digestive system; bleeding as a result of the walls of the blood vessels being eaten away by the acid; and the blockage of the pylorus (the stomach exit) because of the body's attempt to form connective tissue above the ulcer and because of the swelling of the stomach wall in the area of the ulcer.

When we encounter a client with pains in the epigastrium – with or without radiation to the back or behind the sternum – accompanied by heartburn, aggravated before or after food, and relieved by antacids, he must be sent for gastroscopic tests without delay. It is vital to remember that an accurate diagnosis is essential in such situations – when the first complaints occur – in order to negate the possibility of stomach cancer. Thirty percent of stomach cancer cases are discovered as a result of complaints that are reminiscent of an ulcer.

Treatment of ulcers requires medical intervention. However, one of the most important aspects of the treatment is to first remove any factor that intensifies the client's complaint: mental stress, smoking, and so on. By using essential oils, it is possible to help alleviate the pains and balance the client's mental state, which will greatly relieve his pain and will help prevent the ulcer from deteriorating. Moreover, it is important to recommend that the client: (1) maintain a balanced diet according to his body's needs; (2) refrain from eating just before going to sleep, in order to prevent the increased production of stomach acid during sleep; (3) avoid drinking coffee, beverages containing caffeine, decaffeinated coffee, and alcohol; and (4) refrain from eating spicy foods such as red or black pepper, chili powder or any other food that causes him pain and discomfort. In principle, there is no justification in refraining from a particular type of food or beverage unless it is absolutely certain that they are the cause of the discomfort.

Max, a 54-year-old man, the owner of a building supplies factory, came to me because of severe ulcer pains. He underwent a gastroscopic exam that confirmed that he was indeed suffering from a stomach ulcer, and since he was well aware of the dietary implications, he refrained from drinking alcohol, and had recently quit smoking as well. Although he took antacids (the pains often occurred during the day) they only reduced the pain, and he still suffered from severe pains in the epigastrium. The pains caused him to be irritable and intolerant, disrupted the normal course of his work, and much suffering.

During our interview, it was very important for me to focus on Max's mental state. Indeed, as I expected, Max is a man who is under great pressure. It is not easy to avoid being stressed when you are the director of a company that employs many people, when you have to fill customers' orders on time, when you have been hit by the economic recession, and when you are the father of four. However, Max had to understand that his perpetual state of tension plus his nature – to become stressed out easily, to do everything quickly, to work around the clock and not permit himself to rest occasionally – aggravated the state of the ulcer and exacerbated the pains. In addition, Max tended to get upset and angry easily, and when he became irritable, he felt the pains more acutely.

For Max's treatment, I chose oils that alleviate stomach pains and at the same time help calm body and mind in general.

In order to prepare the blend of carrier oils, I used 15 cc of **sunflower** oil (cold-pressed, not the oil used for cooking), 10 cc of **olive** oil (which is known for its superb action on stomach pains in general and on ulcer pains in particular), and 5 cc of **wheatgerm** oil, which is generally excellent for problems of the digestive system. Of the essential oils, I chose **angelica**, which is wonderful for treating many problems of the digestive system, and very effective in alleviating ulcer pains. Moreover, it is a very soothing oil. I dripped five drops of **angelica** into the blend. The second essential oil I used was, of course, **chamomile**. **Chamomile** oil is excellent for a broad range of stomach pains and problems of the digestive system, greatly relieves ulcer pains, and is wonderfully soothing. This oil would help Max calm down, since he suffered from hypersensitivity, irritation, restlessness, stress, and tension. I added five drops of it to the blend. The last oil I chose was **lemon**, which also helps treat ulcer problems, since it assists in creating a base environment in the digestive system. I added five drops of **lemon** to the blend as well.

It is important to point out that the above amounts of essential oil may vary according to the company that produces the oil and its strength.

The three oils I chose are strong oils with dominant odors, and the best way to prepare the blend is to drip them alternately while smelling the blend and making sure that none of the odors dominates. No more than 15 drops of essential oil may be added to an amount of 30 cc of carrier oil. Regarding **lemon** oil, it is important that it not be exposed to the sun for 12 hours after the massage. For this reason, the massage should be performed in the evening, before the person goes to sleep.

In addition, I prepared a pure blend of the essential oils in a 10-cc bottle for Max, for use in an oil burner. When preparing this blend, it is important to balance the oils according to the odor produced by their combination. Although this blend is used primarily for relaxation, and additional or other oils can be used in it (instead of **lemon** oil, since **chamomile** and **angelica** are absolutely vital from the point of view of their relaxing effect in this case), it is always preferable not to "confuse" the person by using a wide range of essential oils. Moreover, it is advisable to use the same oils in a burner as were used in the massage, unless the massage oils are not effective in treating the mental aspect of the problem (which is rare when the choice of oils is holistic).

I asked Max to perform a gentle abdominal massage, using circular movements, for 15-30 minutes each evening, and advised him to go to sleep directly afterwards – or, failing that, to rest or engage in some kind of calm activity that did not require any effort, such as watching TV (nothing that could agitate him) or reading a book.

I asked him to use the oil burner every day, several times a day, especially during work. He was to pour a bit of water – preferably mineral water – into the top saucer of the burner, and add 7-8 drops of the pure essential oil blend (without carrier oils).

Max followed my instructions to the letter. He felt that the massage induced a pleasant, warming, and soothing sensation, and that his stomach pains were significantly relieved afterwards. He discovered that when he performed the massage before going to sleep, he felt much better during the night, slept calmly and peacefully, without being interrupted by discomfort or pain. Moreover, he also woke up with a better feeling in the morning. He used the burner two or three times a day, and even placed a burner in his office. He felt far calmer and more comfortable during the day, and therefore had significant relief from the pains. After two weeks, during which he greatly enjoyed the results of the treatment, I suggested that he reduce the frequency of the massage to three times a week, and after a month, to twice a week. He could continue with that for a long time, if he felt the need for it.

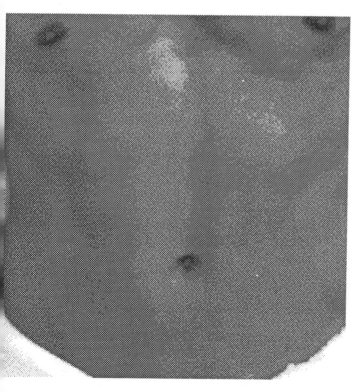

Stomach pain resulting from flatulence

Marla, a high-school teacher of 45 and mother of three, came for aromatherapy because of an annoying and embarrassing problem. She had been suffering from stomach pains and flatulence for a long time as a result of the accumulation of gas in her digestive tract, a problem that also caused her general discomfort and embarrassment. Although she was familiar with various medications for treating flatulence, she did not want to solve the problem by using chemical means, but preferred to try a natural way first. While I was questioning her, I first inquired whether Marla suffered from any allergies to or intolerance of food. As far as she knew, she did not. She tried to eat regular, balanced meals, avoiding legumes, cauliflower, and fried foods, since they intensified the problem acutely. After eating legumes, she would experience very severe stomach pains.

When treating stomach pains resulting from the accumulation of gas in the digestive tract – a very common complaint among all segments of the population – it must be remembered that this problem stems mainly from: some degree of defective digestion; excessive toxins in the digestive tract; eating certain foodstuffs such as legumes, cauliflower, radish, or fried foods. It can sometimes also be a side-effect of constipation, fast eating, or mental stress, and it can stem from an allergy to or intolerance of certain foodstuffs. When treating this problem, the state of the digestive tract must be examined in general to see whether it is necessary to improve the balance of the intestinal flora by taking tablets that contain "friendly" bacteria (such as L. Acidophilus, L. Buligricus, L. Bifadus, and so on). We must also check if the client is allergic to any food and have him refrain from eating foods that cause gas to accumulate in the digestive tract.

Marla actually took food supplements that contained L. Acidophilus for three months, and while she felt a certain relief, the problem was not yet solved. She still suffered from pains and flatulence, mainly two or three hours after eating. During the day, she felt gas forming, which, of course, was very unpleasant for her.

Together with the tablets containing friendly bacteria and the nutritional change in her daily diet, a massage with essential oils would help alleviate the pains, the gas, and the flatulence.

I prepared the following blend for Marla: I poured 25 cc of **almond** and 5 cc of **wheatgerm** oil into a 30-cc bottle. I chose to treat her problem using **fennel** essential oil, which is one of the most important oils for treating the digestive system, since it strengthens it, soothes it, catalyzes its action if it is sluggish, reinforces peristalsis, and helps in cases of accumulation of gas in the tract. Since **fennel** oil is considered to be relatively strong, I only added three drops of it to the blend. I then added six drops of **laurel** essential oil, which is a soothing and warming oil that is beneficial to the digestive system, and three drops of **cardamon** essential oil, which is a stimulating and warming oil that helps many digestive problems, among them that of the accumulation of gases. It is important to note that these three oils are potent, and are not recommended for the treatment of children. Moreover, **fennel** and **laurel** oil are forbidden for use on pregnant women. (The oils that are suitable for treating children with problems of accumulation of gas can be found in the section that deals with this in children and infants.)

Marla was asked to perform a gentle, 15-minute massage of her abdomen once a day for the first week, when she felt that the problem was especially bothering her. She was to perform the massage three times during the second week. Gradually, she would perform the massage only when necessary – when she felt stomach pains as a result of the accumulation of gas.

Marla performed the massage daily for the first week, and followed the nutritional instructions to change her diet. In parallel, she continued taking the tablets containing the friendly bacteria. The massage with essential oils afforded her significant relief, and the stomach pains calmed down and diminished soon after the massage. In addition, she experienced relief from the formation of gas and flatulence. During the second week of treatment, she performed the massage three times, but not on a regular basis – only when she felt pain. Gradually, the pains became less frequent, as did the feeling of the formation and accumulation of gas. The nutritional treatment together with the abdominal massage every time she felt the accumulation of gases, lessened the occurance of stomach pains within a few months, and Marla only needed an abdominal massage once a week – and that only if she felt any discomfort in her digestive tract.

Constipation

Constipation is defined as a condition in which bowel movements are difficult, and the stomach does not work on a regular basis. Like diarrhea, constipation is a relative term, and there are many differences of opinion regarding the normal number of bowel movements per week. In principle, this problem must be dealt with on an individual basis. When a person feels that his weekly bowel movements are fewer than usual, and he feels bloated and has stomach pain, gas, or a general unpleasant physical feeling or heaviness, his condition can be defined as constipation. In any event, when there are three or less bowel movements per week, this is not a normal situation, and even if the person feels fine, a state of excessive toxins in his digestive tract and intestines can occur, and this can go on for many years. Gradually, this state can damage his digestive system, and his body may become debilitated and its functions jeopardized to some extent.

The constipation that is common, generally stems from incorrect intestinal habits that result from nutrition. Both the absence of a sufficient amount of dietary fiber in food and an insufficient amount of liquids are considered to be significant causes of constipation. Another cause of constipation is too small an amount of fats in the diet. Similarly, constipation can be a side-effect of other problems and of many different causes such as: various diseases that cause a partial blockage of the intestinal opening (tumors, for instance), constipation that occurs as a reaction to various inflammations of the anus or hemorrhoids (when the person might fear the pain during evacuation), nervous disorders in the intestinal movement, diseases of the intestinal muscle, time pressure or change of place, mental disorders such as depression, and so on.

Essential oils are very effective in the treatment of constipation. In conjunction with aromatherapy, it is important to see that the person eats at fixed times in order to get the intestines accustomed to a daily bowel movement, usually at the same time, in a comfortable, unhurried way. When the person is acutely constipated and bowel movements become painful and irksome, or when there is anal pain, it is a good idea for him to take his mind off the bowel movement by reading a newspaper or listening to the radio. However, it must be remembered that in cases of recurring anal fissures, he must see that his bowel movements are very short, and he must not linger in the bathroom.

It is very important to eat a lot of vegetables and dietary fiber in order to increase the volume of the feces. In this way, the bowel movement reflex becomes more effective.

Regular physical exercise is essential when there is constipation, and if exercise is lacking, it can cause constipation. This can be overcome by a daily walk or any other daily physical exercise.

In addition, it is important to drink a lot – a small amount of the liquid is not absorbed, and helps soften the lumps of food residues that enter the intestine, increases their volume, and helps move them along the large intestine. It is also important to check whether there is an insufficient consumption of fats, and add accordingly, since the effect of fats on the feces is similar to that of water.

In every client with secondary or reactionary constipation (that is, constipation resulting from a particular disease or problem), it is necessary to discover the reasons for it and deal with them accordingly. Essential oils must also be matched holistically to the sum total of the problems from which the person suffers – the primary problem and the problem of constipation itself. In clients whose constipation is a reaction to inflamed hemorrhoids and pain, the treatment must focus on the hemorrhoids, with local ointments, suppositories for alleviating the pain, and substances to soften the feces (prescribed by a physician) to prevent pain during the bowel movement. Moreover, a sitz bath containing essential oils or suitable herbal infusions should be taken in order to solve the problem of hemorrhoids. When constipation is a result of a mental problem, the problem must be treated inclusively and holistically, using the appropriate essential oils. Depression, which is frequently accompanied by secondary constipation, must be treated with antidepressant essential oils (see the section on depression). In cases of constipation, it is possible to consume fibers via foods that are rich in them, such as oat bran fibers and guar gum. In this case, the client must see that he drinks enough and ensure that the increased consumption of fiber does not create dietary deficits in his body (fibers tend to absorb various vitamins and minerals and excrete them from the body).

Jesse came for treatment of chronic constipation from which he had been suffering for several years. Jesse was a big man in his late 60s who, until recently, had not paid any attention to his eating habits or to his physical health. Before retiring, he had never been ill, except for the odd cold or bout of flu. He had owned a welding factory, where he himself worked along with several employees. After a cup of coffee, a cigarette, and a cookie, he would leave home early in the morning and work long hours in his factory. He sometimes even skipped his lunch break, or he would spend it with one of his workmates over a cup of coffee. Frequently, his dinner was the first full meal he had eaten the whole day. Accordingly, this was a heavy meal that contained a large quantity of meat. When he was still working, the physical work compensated for the physical damage that occurred as a result of his incorrect nutrition. Moreover, his work environment and his commitment to it were incentives for him to immerse himself entirely in his work, and did not leave him much time to focus on himself. When he retired, having sold the factory, Jesse found himself with nothing to do, and with very few interests. He found himself sitting in front of the TV for hours. While he enjoyed his freedom and the chance to spend a lot of time with his wife, his grown-up children, and his first grandchild, the lack of physical activity soon took its toll, since his eating habits had not changed, except that he now ate additional meals...

He put on some weight, but what mainly bothered him was the change in the frequency of his bowel movements. Before retiring, he had never had a problem with constipation, but the change in his lifestyle caused a situation in which he was now suffering from ongoing constipation – to the point that he sometimes only had a bowel movement every three or four days. This made him feel bloated, gave his stomach a "swollen" appearance, created gas, and caused an unpleasant feeling.

Another disturbing thing he mentioned while I was interviewing him was that he felt that his memory and his powers of concentration had deteriorated slightly since he had stopped working.

As part of the combined treatment, which included, of course, balanced nutrition and a program of appropriate physical exercise, Jesse was treated with essential oils.

In such a case, the oils have a tremendous advantage. The change in nutrition, the addition of dietary fibers, and physical exercise would probably speed up and balance the action of Jesse's intestines. However, those changes, especially at his age, could take a long time, and the results would not always be quick. In the meantime, before the problem was solved, the client could suffer acutely from the symptoms that made him come for treatment in the first place – constipation. This is where the essential oils play an important role. Aromatherapy is a holistic treatment in which we not only focus on oils for treating constipation, but also match the oils to the client's problems and character. In addition, the oils help speed up and balance the client's peristalsis, support his digestive tract, soothe flatulence and stomach pains, and noticeably speed up bowel movements. Remember that it is always important to focus on the holistic treatment of a number of aspects in order to achieve good and lasting results.

The essential oils that are generally recommended for treating constipation are **basil**, **fennel** (for the general treatment of the digestive tract), **camphor**, **orange** (good for chronic constipation), **marjoram**, **yarrow**, **rosemary**, and **lemon**.

The first essential oil I chose for Jesse's treatment was **rosemary**, which is an excellent oil for encouraging intestinal movement, and would also stimulate Jesse's mind, thus helping to solve his memory and concentration problems. The next oil was **fennel**, which strengthens the peristalsis, helps in cases of constipation, stimulates the action of the digestive system in general, and even helps balance the appetite, which was important in Jesse's case.

I dripped 10 drops of **rosemary** oil and five drops of **fennel** oil into 30 cc of **grapeseed** carrier oil. I asked Jesse to massage his abdomen with the blend for 15 minutes, using gentle clockwise movements, once in the morning and once in the evening.

During the first days of treatment, Jesse did not feel any improvement in his condition, but after a week of massage, he began to feel better, and had a larger number of bowel movements than usual. His bowel movements were not yet as regular as they should have been, but there was a great improvement. Jesse told me that good bowel movements helped him stick to his new dietary habits and to the regimen of physical exercise that had been devised for him. Initially, because of his heavy and bloated feeling, he did not feel like exercising. He also reported an improvement in his mood and a much better feeling in his abdomen.

About two weeks later, during which time Jesse administered self-massage and took supplements of dietary fiber, along with sticking to his new diet, his bowel movements began to be increasingly regular and easy, and the bloated feeling began to decrease. After a few months of this combined treatment and his twice-daily massage, his bowel movements became regular on a daily basis, and his general condition and feeling improved beyond recognition. He felt more alert, lighter, and even calmer, and now that he was trying to do some physical exercise during the day and to eat correctly, his constipation problems became a thing of the past, and his digestive tract functioned much more efficiently.

Mouth ulcers

Jean, a geriatric nurse of 52, sat beside me in one of the lectures I attended. During the break, when she heard me talk a little about aromatherapy, she asked for some quick, simple, and effective advice for treating a minor but annoying problem. She had been suffering from small mouth ulcers for years. They appeared, lasted for a few days – sometimes for over a week – then slowly disappeared. The ulcers were very painful, especially when she ate, and because they sometimes protruded, she bit them while chewing, and then the pain was acute.

Mouth ulcers, a common problem that afflicts many people, are tears or cuts in the inner covering of the mouth, and are generally felt when eating spicy or acidic food. They look like a yellowish or whitish dot surrounded by a bright redness. While they are generally small, they sometimes occur in clusters and are extremely painful. They usually disappear naturally in a week or two.

There are two very common types of mouth ulcers. When treating ulcers with holistic therapy or aromatherapy, the type of ulcer and its causes must be taken into account.

Fungal ulcers – the painful and annoying type – are liable to occur during periods of pressure, stress, and depression, or as a side-effect of a disease. They may be caused by a virus or when the immune system is particularly weak. (It is important to check this, especially when the ulcers recur frequently.) Ulcers of this type are very common among adolescents and pre-adolescents, and they are more common in women, especially before menstruation.

The second type, which is just as painful, is the ulcer that is caused by damage to the inner covering of the mouth as a result of eating very hot food, brushing teeth, biting the skin, and so on.

It is possible to treat the ulcer itself quickly and effectively with aromatherapy. Having said that, the symptomatic treatment offered below notwithstanding, it is very important to check out the following in cases of ulcers that recur frequently at brief intervals: Did the ulcer occur after a disease? Did it occur as a result of a bite or damage to the mouth? Is the person going through a period of great pressure, depression or stress (or has he just been through such a period)?

Moreover, it is important to check the state of the immune system (is the person prone to infections, yeast infections, many infectious winter diseases and so on?), the state of the hormonal system (are there additional indications of a lack of balance – irregular periods, acne, endocrine problems, and so on?), and whether the person suffers from any allergies or food intolerance.

Frequently recurring mouth ulcers often provide us with a clue to the person's general condition, and, accordingly, he can be given an inclusive treatment that deals with all the problems and can solve the occurance of mouth ulcers completely.

Since Jean asked for a symptomatic treatment for the problem, I recommended that she take a cotton-tipped swab and drip two drops of pure, undiluted **clove** or **tea tree** oil onto it. Using the swab, she was to apply the oil gently to every ulcer several times a day. If her saliva mixed with the oils, she was to spit it out and not swallow it.

Jean tried the treatment using **tea tree** oil and, very shortly after applying it, her mouth ulcers shrank and healed. Within a few days, she no longer felt them at all.

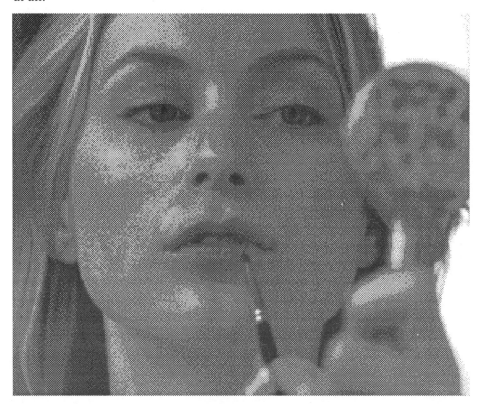

Oral herpes

Trish, a 17-year-old high-school student, wanted to try aromatherapy in order to solve a problem that had been plaguing her for a long time. She asked for an effective and immediate treatment for herpes, which broke out every now and then, surrounding her lips with ugly sores. Trish's herpes outbreaks occurred mainly during the winter, and caused her unnecessary embarrassment. Unnecessary, because there is really nothing to be ashamed of. Herpes is a common disease, and although it can also break out on the genitals and be transferred during sexual contact, this does not necessarily attest to how it was contracted.

Herpes is a rash of blisters that is caused by the viral infection *herpes simplex*. After the virus has been contracted, the infection can lie dormant in the nervous system, and break out as a result of exposure to cold or heat, a respiratory tract infection, menstruation, a viral infection such as flu, an emotional crisis, or a mental trauma. The outbreak of the disease is manifested in sores around the mouth, and sometimes also on the genitals. The disease is contagious, and this should be taken into account.

Nowadays, there are various medications used for treating the signs of the outbreak, but there are still no preparations that prevent the disease entirely. It is possible to feel the beginning of an outbreak by itching and prickling sensations in the area, and the sores tend to disappear after about a week.

Trish asked for a natural, safe, and immediate solution, but since we are talking about herpes, it is not always possible to expect appreciable success. Aromatherapy often helps relieve the irritation, alleviate the state of the sores somewhat, and even shorten their duration. However, only when we treat the problem as part of an inclusive treatment of the person's state of health and mind – a treatment that combines aspects of strengthening the immune system and strengthening the mental and emotional aspect – is it possible to avoid an outbreak, especially when aromatherapy constitutes a part of the combined holistic treatment. When treating the herpes sores themselves or when the person feels that they are about to occur, **lavender** or **tea tree** oils in their pure form must be applied locally, directly onto the skin, and only on the specific area, using a cotton-tipped swab. These two oils are highly recommended, since their low toxicity permits their undiluted (neat) application.

Using a swab, one of the following oils can also be applied locally to each sore: **chamomile, lemon, geranium,** and **bergamot**. However, in this case, I recommend applying a drop of the oil to the hand or to the inside of the arm in order to see how the skin reacts to it (especially in the case of **bergamot**, which must always be checked before use), waiting a few hours, and applying it to the sore only if no irritation has occurred.

When we treat herpes as a secondary problem resulting from a more major problem, we also include soothing oils, antiviral oils, and oils for strengthening the immune system in the general treatment. Oils that lower a fever can also be effective in the blend. (Especially suitable, for other purposes too, are **eucalyptus**, which is suitable in general for treating herpes, **melissa**, the oil that has an effect on the emotional aspect, and can be appropriate in such cases, or **chamomile**, which also has an excellent effect on the emotional aspect.)

When Trish applied pure **lavender** oil to the sores several times a day, the burning and irritation decreased, and there was an improvement in the appearance of the sores. The duration of the sores was shorter than before, but she could not attribute the improvement solely to the treatment, since she had already experienced changes in the duration of the sores in the past.

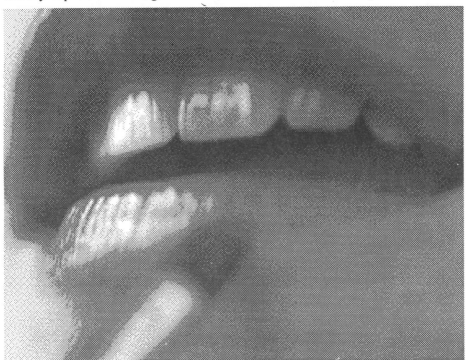

Joint diseases (arthritis and rheumatism)

Joint diseases are among the most common diseases for which essential oils are used as support treatment. These diseases can be ongoing and painful, and sometimes involve great mental suffering, as well as an inability to perform various physical activities. Treatment with essential oils provides the client with great relief from physical pain and emotional suffering, and often brings about an improvement in his condition, when it is administered professionally and over a long time, and especially when it is part of a combined holistic treatment.

There are various types of joint diseases and inflammations, and, when a client comes for aromatherapy or wants to treat himself with essential oils, it is important to identify which kind he is suffering from, and use the appropriate essential oils.

In general, the essential oils used for joint diseases are anti-inflammatory, soothing, disinfectant, and liquid-absorbing oils. When it is bacterial arthritis, antibacterial oils must be added to the blend, and when it is viral arthritis, antiviral oils must be added. Among the essential oils that are generally recommended for treating these diseases are **lavender** (which is anti-inflammatory, antiviral, antibacterial, soothing, and strengthens the immune system), **cypress**, **juniper**, **eucalyptus**, **marjoram**, **camphor** (not for general massage, and not for prolonged use), **clary sage**, **niaouli**, **yarrow**, **chamomile**, and **bergamot** (which are also anti-inflammatory). **Benzoin**, **tea tree**, **peppermint**, **cajeput**, **rosemary**, and **thyme** are generally effective in soothing and relieving joint pains.

Sandra, a 45-year-old mother of three and a bank clerk by profession, had been suffering from rheumatoid arthritis for three years. Rheumatoid arthritis is a systemic disease whose cause is unknown. It can focus on the synovial membranes of the joint and/or cause many extra-joint complications.

The disease tends mainly to affect the hands and feet, and the course of the disease is characterized by alternate flare-ups and respites. As a result of the chronic inflammatory process, there is a creation of nuclear tissue (called pannus) that penetrates the neighboring bony organs (bones, cartilage, tendons) and gradually destroys them. Following this, there is advanced destruction of the joint. Unfortunately, in certain cases, the disease can also cause extra-joint phenomena that can include subcutaneous nodosity, inflammation of the blood vessels, neuropathic disorders (disorders in the nerve function), damage to the heart (myocarditis), or damage to the lungs. The causes of the disease are unknown, and some think that it is some kind of immunological process. The process may begin as a result of the body's reaction to a primary stimulus such as an infection, but the reason for the onset of the disease is still not clear.

In Sandra's case, the arthritis appeared in the form of symmetrical polyarthritis. She complained of pain, redness, sensitivity, swelling, and limited movement in the affected joints, which, in her case, were her wrists and knees (the pains were likely to occur in other places too, such as the hips and spine). Sandra's pain was more acute in the morning, after she woke up, and she felt a painful stiffness in the joints. She noted that the acute pain and the stiffness occurred mainly after periods of rest, such as in the afternoon, but diminished and calmed down after some activity.

Other signs that can appear with joint inflammations (Sandra did not suffer from these) are weakness, a lack of appetite, a low-grade fever, and often difficulty in performing routine, everyday actions. Today, Sandra can still perform most everyday actions, and still function normally at work. However, mainly during the morning, these actions are accompanied by severe pain that diminish during the day. In different arthritis patients, there can also be subcutaneous nodosity (especially in the joint region), enlargement of lymph nodes, muscular atrophy (as a result of muscles not being used), and in chronically ill patients, deformation of the joints, tears in the tendons, and infections in the spine.

Sandra's condition was considered to be relatively good with regard to the gravity of the disease, and this could be attributed mostly to the fact that she did not succumb to the disease, but tried to move and be active. This kept her muscles from weakening and atrophying.

As a rule, regular physical exercise is highly recommended for people suffering from joint diseases. It is advisable for them to get suitable advice about the most appropriate physical exercise for their particular condition. Moreover, obesity is one of the causes of increased pressure on the joints, so it is important to maintain correct and healthy eating habits and the correct weight.

The acute stage of the disease is treated with anti-inflammatory drugs that do not belong to the corticosteroid group. These drugs include: aspirin, brufen, voltaren, etc. Most of these drugs have a similar effect in relieving pain and halting the inflammatory process. For patients who do not respond to this treatment, special injections are considered. Some try treatment that affects the immune system. The treatment with corticosteroids, which has many side effects, is reserved for special cases with complications that do not respond to the rest of the treatments. In parallel to treatment with medications, suitable physiotherapy must be administered in order to prevent, as much as possible, contractural deformations (a state of a lack of nutrition in the joint as a result of a lack of pliancy in the structures around it), and in order to afford the patient maximum movement despite the disease. Although the disease is chronic and causes prolonged suffering, it does not shorten the life span and, in fact, may decline over the years and enter a phase of minimal activity. Therefore treatments that cause severe side-effects are to be avoided (such as exaggerated treatment with corticosteroids). Having said that, it is possible to inject corticosteroids into the joint in certain cases. Moreover, orthopedic surgery offers successful operations for correcting deformations, sometimes to the point of replacing entire joints with artificial ones.

In addition, it is important to ensure that the client receives the appropriate nutrition. While we are not aware of a specific menu or specific ingredients that can improve conditions of rheumatoid arthritis with absolute certainty, there are some that may well reduce some of the symptoms of the disease, such as stiffening of the limbs and pains. Therefore, it is important to consult with an orthomolecular therapist or a dietician. It has been found that there are cases in which the arthritis is accompanied by an allergy to certain foods, that is, by the production of antibodies against one of the ingredients. It is possible that this reaction is what causes the arthritis in these cases. There are reports of cases in which abstinence from allergy-causing foods – such as dairy products, wheat products, eggs, and soya – alleviated the illness. Identifying the allergenic factor and removing it from the patient's menu may significantly improve his condition. Thus, it is important to undergo special allergy treatment in order to discover the foods that cause allergies.

It has been found that the fatty acid, Omega 3, which is found in North Sea fish, weakens the arthritic process. The fatty acid, linoleic gamma (Omega 6), operates in a similar way to Omega 3, since it causes a decrease in the production of the icosanoids that increase the arthritic reaction. This acid is found in the oils produced from evening primrose, from the seeds of wild black raspberries, and from the foxtail plant. Moreover, a zinc supplement can reduce some of the symptoms of the disease. The carrier oils that contain high levels of linoleic gamma fatty acid can bring relief to arthritis sufferers, so it is important to include them in an aromatherapy treatment.

Sandra was being treated by a nutrition and allergy specialist, but this treatment would go on for a few years, and in the meantime she wanted some kind of treatment that would help alleviate her pains, the stiffness in her joints, the redness, and the swelling.

With aromatherapy, there are many oils that are suitable for treating arthritis and joint pains. Among the essential oils that are suitable for rheumatism are **cajeput, eucalyptus, angelica, lavender, rosemary, juniper, lemon, marjoram, chamomile, yarrow, cinnamon, niaouli, ginger**, and **thyme**. For treating joint pains in general, **benzoin, tea tree, peppermint**, and **camphor** oils can be used. (**Camphor** must not be used for a general massage, nor for a prolonged period of time. Although it is suitable for treating joint pains, it has a high level of toxicity, and so a different oil should be chosen.)

The treatment I prepared for Sandra consisted of three stages: a bath, a body massage that focused on the damaged joints, and a local massage of the painful joints to be performed by Sandra herself. The first stage was the bath. This helps relieve pain and alleviate the stiffness in the joints. The bath is a salt bath – the essential oils are dissolved in a tablespoon of salt before being placed in the warm bath water. I asked Sandra to drip one drop each of **cypress, lavender**, and **juniper** oils onto the salt. She was to fill the bath with pleasantly warm water, mix the spoon of salt and essential oils into it, and remain in the water for a long time – up to an hour. If the water cooled down, hot water could be added carefully in order to maintain the warm temperature of the water. I asked Sandra to take advantage of the time in the bath in order to relax. Also, to prevent her from becoming bored during her long soak, I recommended that she put on pleasant, soothing music, and become accustomed to abdominal breathing exercises for three to five minutes. While she was in the bath, it was a good idea for her to massage and rub the stiff joints a bit, and move them in circular movements.

During the first week, I recommended the bath treatment for Sandra on a daily basis. During the second week, when massage was added three times a week, she was to take the bath on alternate days – that is, a bath on the days she was not having a massage. In the third week, she should take only three baths, and from the second month of treatment onward, only two baths a week, continuing in this way for several months.

Sandra began the bath treatment. She reported that after the bath, which she took prior to going to sleep, she felt much better. Her joints were still stiff, red, and swollen, but there was some relief in the stiffness and swelling, as well as in the level of pain. However, in the morning, the pain was as severe as ever, and no improvement was evident.

At this point, we moved on to the second stage of the treatment – massage with essential oils. We performed the massage three times during the first week, and on those days, there was no need for her to take a bath. For the massage, I chose to treat Sandra with the following oils: 15 cc of **almond** oil (**grapeseed** oil can also be used), 5 cc of **evening primrose** oil (this can be omitted, and then 20 cc of **almond** or **grapeseed** oil must be used), 5 cc of **jojoba** oil, and 5 cc of **wheatgerm** oil. Of the essential oils, I chose to add five drops of **cajeput** oil, which is very effective in the treatment of joint pains, a powerful disinfectant, warming and stimulating; five drops of **ginger** oil, which is also warming and stimulating, and excellent for treating rheumatism; and **rosemary** oil, which is a powerful disinfectant, analgesic, warming, invigorating, and suitable for treating arthritis. As we can see, the massage blend included mainly warming, invigorating and stimulating oils, while the bath blend was more soothing.

The massage was administered to Sandra's entire body for almost an hour, while concentrating on the stiff and painful areas with a warming and invigorating massage. After the massage, Sandra felt immediate relief in the stiffness in her joints, and the relief continued until the next day.

I gave Sandra an identical blend of carrier and essential oils to take home, and asked her to perform a massage on the stiff areas twice a day – if possible, when she got up in the morning, before going to work, in order to relieve the severe morning pains, and at night. She was to perform this massage every day.

About a week later, during which Sandra had four baths on the days she did not have a general body massage, and received three general massages (and made sure to massage the painful joints for 15 minutes at least twice a day), Sandra reported a significant improvement in the stiffness and pain in her joints. Moreover, she mentioned that there seemed to be an additional decrease in the swelling of her joints.

Sandra was meticulous about administering the treatments. In the second week of massage treatment, we went down to two general massages a week for two months, and after seeing an additional improvement in her condition as well as in the state of redness and swelling of the joints, and a decrease in the morning pains, too, we went down to one general massage a week for a few months, while Sandra made sure to administer the local massages and take baths.

The aromatherapy did not solve Sandra's problem entirely. She still suffers from stiffness in the joints, and sometimes from severe pain, too. However, she feels a great relief in the pain, swelling, and redness in the joints, and reports a decrease in the stiffness. This relief helps her function much better during the day. The supportive treatment helps her to a great extent, especially at times when the disease flares up and the pain becomes almost unbearable, and then the massage and the baths are of great help in decreasing the pain level and enabling her to return to her normal, everyday functioning.

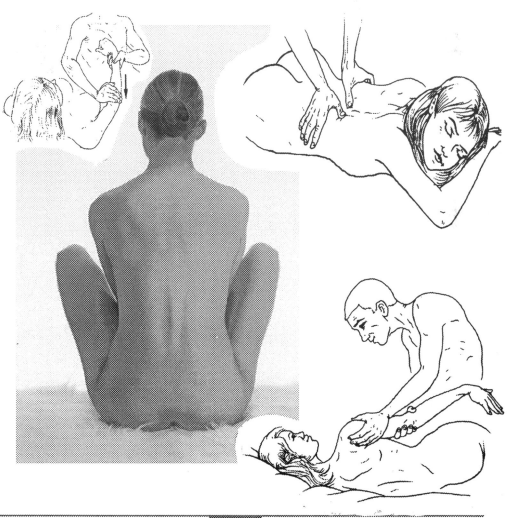

Another form of inflammation of the joint is bacterial arthritis, in which we use slightly different oils, taking into account the fact that bacterial arthritis has different causes. Most of the cases are caused by bacteria in the blood circulation. It can occur as a result of environmental pollution infection. Thus, when treating this disease with aromatherapy, we use mainly antibacterial oils such as **lemon, tea tree, thyme, petitgrain, lavender** and **niaouli**, which are recommended principally in states of low vitality. In addition, it is very important to reinforce the immune system with suitable oils, because the seriousness of the diseases can increase as the immune system grows weaker. **Bergamot, lavender, lemon, tea tree**, and **chamomile** oils, which we use for other aspects of the diseases, are oils that greatly reinforce the action of the immune system.

Bacterial arthritis generally occurs in one joint, but it can also occur in several different joints. Using essential oils, we massage the client's entire body, diluting the oils, determining the duration of the treatment according to the client's level of vitality, and concentrating on the affected joints.

In order to identify whether it really is a case of bacterial arthritis, a physician must be consulted. The disease is diagnosed by drawing liquid from the affected joint, and finding an increased number of cells, low concentrations of glucose, and the presence of bacteria in the direct swab and in the culture. The medical treatment generally includes large amounts of intravenous antibiotics, and aromatherapy does not interfere with it, but rather relieves the pain and improves the client's general functioning.

The treatment of bacterial arthritis is similar to the treatment of other joint inflammations – aromatic baths, general and local massage – except that in this case, as we said before, we include antibacterial oils in the blend of oils for treating these diseases. The blend for the bath can contain one drop of **lavender** oil, which reinforces the immune system (and is also suitable for treating arthritis) because of its antibacterial and anti-inflammatory properties; one drop of **lemon** oil, which, besides being suitable for treating joint pains and arthritis, is also a powerful antibacterial oil; and one drop of **chamomile** oil, which is anti-inflammatory and suitable for treating arthritis, and reinforces the immune system. Of course, it is important to take the bath in the evening, before going to sleep, since the **lemon** oil is phototoxic, and must not be exposed to sunlight for about 12 hours after being applied.

The massage blend can consist of five drops of **thyme** oil for adults, or **sweet thyme** (for children or people with a low level of vitality), which are oils that help in the treatment of arthritis and are, additionally, antibacterial and disinfectant oils; five drops of **tea tree** oil, which is an extremely powerful antibacterial oil, as well as being a powerful disinfectant; and five drops of **cajeput** oil, using the same carrier oils as in the treatment of non-bacterial joint inflammations.

The general body massage should be administered three times during the first week, as necessary, and possibly during the second week as well (when the client's vitality is normal; a client with low vitality should undergo shorter massages less frequently), and is reduced to two massages during the second or third week, and to one or two in the following weeks, according to the extent of improvement in his condition.

We ask the client or his family to administer the local massage every day, twice a day, for about 15 minutes.

If the client's vitality is low, the duration of the massage is shorter.

As a rule, the guiding principle in treating bacterial arthritis, as opposed to regular arthritis, is adding antibacterial oils to the treatment blend.

Back pains

Barry, a 45-year-old semitrailer driver, came for aromatherapy because of a very common complaint. After working as a truck driver for over 15 years, Barry suffered from the most common problem experienced by his colleagues – back pains. Although he had been using a special orthopedic seat for years, and this relieved his pain somewhat, he still felt as if his back was going to break when he came home after an eight-hour driving shift.

Back pains are a very common problem, and the possible causes are vast. These causes range from working long hours while standing, wearing high-heeled shoes, and doing hard physical labor, through bad posture, slipped disks, and serious vertebral problems. For this reason, when a client is suffering from back pains, the first thing to do is to diagnose the cause of the pains, and this is not easy. When there are serious pains for unknown causes, it is advisable to refrain from administering treatment before ascertaining what the problem is, in order not to cause damage. When the pain is caused by external factors, such as prolonged walking in high-heeled shoes, hard labor, and so on, aromatherapy is very effective in alleviating it. Aromatherapy with massage and baths considerably improves the client's condition, helps relax tense muscles, and relieves pain.

Many oils can be used for treating back and muscle pains. Among them are **black pepper**, **rosemary**, **chamomile**, **cajeput**, **eucalyptus**, **lavender**, **basil**, **tea tree**, **marjoram**, **peppermint**, **camphor**, **niaouli** (which is suitable for muscle and back pains in children), **thyme**, **pine**, **wintergreen**, **benzoin** (especially for muscle spasms), **lemongrass** (especially for muscle spasms), **laurel** and **nutmeg**. Some of these oils are analgesic (see the chapter on treatment with essential oils in sensitive conditions), and by anesthetizing the nerve endings, the pains are alleviated to a large extent.

For Barry's treatment, I chose to use the following oils for a bath: one drop of analgesic **lavender** oil, which alleviates pains; one drop of **black pepper** oil, which is analgesic, antispasmodic, and extremely effective in the treatment of back pains and muscle spasms; one drop of **pine** oil, which is excellent for treating back and muscle pains; and one drop of **nutmeg** oil, which is also analgesic, antispasmodic, and very effective in treating muscle pains. I suggested that Barry take a nice, warm, soothing bath when he got home from work, and stay in it for about 20 minutes.

In addition, it is very advisable to undergo massage. Since Barry had told me that his wife had "golden hands," and would be happy to massage his back and do as much as she could to help treat his back pains, the massage treatment was assigned to her capable hands. The massage blend that I prepared for Barry contained 10 cc **sunflower** oil (**almond** oil can also be used), two drops of **black pepper** oil, two drops of **laurel** oil, and one drop of **rosemary** oil. (In the hands of an experienced, professional therapist, two drops of **wintergreen** oil can be added. However, this is not the case with self-treatment at home, because of the high level of toxicity of this oil.)

Barry began to take regular baths with aromatic oils, and immediately after the bath, his wife massaged his back, exerting mild pressure (very lovingly!). It is interesting to mention that Barry felt an improvement after the first bath, but felt an increase in pain after the massage – not significant, but evident. This is normal, since sometimes, after the massage, the body gets out of its apparent balance, and the pains are felt more strongly. This is the result of the massage, especially when it is performed with pressure, or as deep massage, and not the result of the essential oils. Since the blend contained analgesic oils, Barry did not feel this change significantly.

After a few treatments, Barry began to feel a decrease in his back pains, even though it was not significant. However, the situation did improve slightly. When he had undergone this treatment for two full weeks, he felt significant and substantial relief. Because this occurred so rapidly, it was decided that he would gradually reduce his treatment to alternating baths and massages, or undergo treatment only when he felt pain.

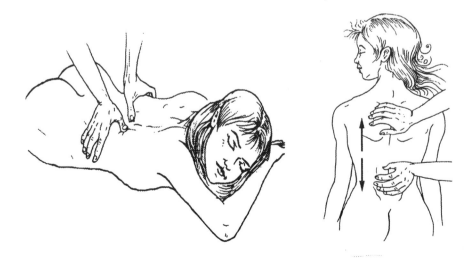

Earache / External ear infections

Brad, the son of close friends, summoned me for "first aid" treatment when he developed a painful ear infection. A few days before, he had had his ear pierced at a rather unsavory place, and now he was paying the price. Of course, he had no choice but to take out the earring, and now his earlobe was red and painful, and swelling was evident around the hole.

When there is an internal ear infection, it is important to obtain medical treatment, since this condition can lead to various complications that are particularly serious in children and adults alike. No risk should be taken.

An external ear or earlobe infection is generally caused by a cut, a sore, or careless piercing. Nose piercing is liable to cause a similar infection (not always because of the person who performs the piercing. An infection in the nose as a result of piercing is frighteningly common). As long as the infection is characterized by swelling, pain, and redness, and there is no appearance of pus, it can be treated with essential oils. If there is pus, a suitable antibiotic ointment for treating such infections should be used.

In order to treat the infection in Brad's earlobe, I dipped a cotton-tipped swab in a little **tea tree** oil and applied it to the infected lobe between three and five times a day. I entrusted the remainder of the treatment to Brad, instructing him to apply the oil to his lobe with a cotton-tipped swab between three and five times a day. Of course, he was not allowed to reinsert the earring until long after the infection had disappeared.

In addition to **tea tree** oil, **lavender** and **geranium** oils are also very effective in treating external ear infections. A drop or two of one of the above oils is placed, undiluted, on a cotton bud and applied to the ear several times a day, until the infection disappears.

Brad followed my instructions meticulously, applying the oil to the infected area several times a day. Within a few days, the redness and the swelling disappeared, as did the pain. Brad had to wait a long time before reinserting the earring, which in fact he shouldn't do at all, since in such cases, it is possible that the earlobe is allergic to the earring, and the infection can recur. In any event, when there is an infection as a result of ear piercing, it is absolutely essential that the earring be thoroughly disinfected with alcohol before being reinserted in the ear, and it is advisable to wait until the ear is absolutely healed before reinserting the earring.

Hypertension

The treatment of hypertension should be administered by professional aromatherapists, masseurs, and reflexologists. Novice aromatherapists require the supervision and counseling of an experienced practitioner.

Scott, 68 years old, came for aromatherapy principally because he suffered from high blood pressure. An active retiree who used to be a math teacher, Scott was now working as a volunteer, giving private lessons at the community center near his home. He defined himself as a "strong person." He had never suffered from illnesses or significant pains (even though he had spent many years doing hard physical labor before becoming a teacher).

Now he was complaining of high blood pressure – 150/90 – that was being controlled with medications. Without the medications, his blood pressure would reach 230. Moreover, he had been suffering from weakness and irritability for some time, and now defined himself as a person "who got hot under the collar quickly," and who was very easy to aggravate. He had always been a hot-tempered man, but aging and quitting regular work had made him even more sensitive. He could blow up when something didn't sit right with him – while watching TV or reading the newspaper, when his grown-up children expressed views that he found unacceptable, and so on. In the past, he would flush, shout, argue, and get angry. Now, when his children were themselves parents, he would simply get really mad and leave the room. He would continue to feel angry for long minutes after the incident, and found it hard to calm down.

In addition to his high blood pressure, Scott complained of sleeping difficulties. He slept very lightly, and would wake up at any little sound. However, it was his high blood pressure that was really worrying him.

A point that is important to mention is that when treating clients with hypertension, *the following oils must not be used under any circumstances*: **sage** *and* **red thyme**. Moreover, if **rosemary, cinnamon, camphor** and **sweet thyme** essential oils are used at all, it is only when treating clients whose hypertension is controlled, and must only be administered by an experienced, professional aromatherapist. These oils raise blood pressure and are not recommended for use in such cases. Similarly, the addition of **lavender** oil to a blend whose orientation is to raise blood pressure will enhance this action. For this reason, precautionary measures must be taken, even with people who have only a *tendency* toward high blood pressure. To the same extent, this special property of **lavender** oil is reflected when we use a blend whose orientation is to lower blood pressure; it will enhance this action in the direction of lowering blood pressure. (**Lavender** oil usually enhances the general direction of the blend of oils.)

Treatment with massage and reflexology, which are very effective in the treatment of hypertension, should only be performed by experienced and professional aromatherapists. A person who is not professional should administer treatment with an oil burner only.

For Scott's treatment, I used the following carrier oils: 20 cc **grapeseed** oil, 5 cc **wheatgerm** oil, and 5 cc **evening primrose** oil, which is an oil that helps maintain the blood vessels, regulate blood pressure, expand the blood vessels, and prevent thromboses. I added the following essential oils to a 30-cc bottle of carrier oils: three drops of **lavender** oil, which is known to balance and lower blood pressure, and would also help Scott calm down and reduce his level of stress as a result of its beneficial emotional effects. It would also help a little in improving his sleep. (Another important point is that it is one of the best oils for reinforcing the immune system, which is something we want in every aromatherapy blend). The second oil I chose was **marjoram**. This oil induces a calm, warming, and comforting feeling, and works wonderfully in the treatment of hypertension. It helps the general circulation and expands blood vessels. In addition, it is thought to be a stimulating oil, which is important in balancing an aromatic blend in which there are mainly soothing oils. I placed three drops of **marjoram** oil into the blend, and added two drops of **melissa** oil, which helps lower blood pressure and has soothing effects on the mental state, and three drops of **neroli** oil, which also lowers blood pressure, helps in cases of insomnia, soothes, and moderates the heart rate. As we can see, Scott's massage blend is more diluted than usual because of the especially delicate treatment reserved for people with hypertension.

We do not let clients administer self-massage or undergo "amateur" massages when their blood pressure is not balanced, since we must not take any risks. Of course, we have to find out whether there are any other problems, such as heart disease, kidney disease, and so on, that can rule out treatment by massage. The same goes for a bath. However, as a first step, I prepared a neat blend of essential oils for Scott, for self-use at home – only in an oil burner.

Scott's treatment included an extremely gentle massage once a week for about 35 minutes; a weekly treatment with reflexology and essential oils, including a special method for lowering blood pressure (to be administered by a qualified reflexologist only); treatment with lukewarm baths twice a week for 15 minutes each time; and the use of an oil burner at least twice a day (once around bed-time).

After the first massage treatment, Scott was surprised at how calm and relaxed he felt. At this stage, we did not yet measure the change in his blood pressure, since the process can take a long time, and the change does not necessarily occur immediately after the first treatment (even though there are such cases). The next day, he sat in a bath for about 15 minutes and used the oil burner according to the instructions. The reflexology treatment, which was performed with the same essential oils, gave him a marvelous feeling of power and vitality.

The following week, Scott mentioned that he definitely felt an overall change – from the emotional rather than the physical point of view. He felt far calmer, and as a result did not get upset too much during the week. He still complained of sleeping difficulties, but said that he felt a change for the better.

After three weeks of treatment during which a general improvement in Scott's condition occurred, his physician reported a slight lowering of his blood pressure, which, while signaling a positive trend, did not yet justify any kind of reduction in the dosage of his medications. Scott himself was very pleased with the new feeling of calmness that he had attained and with the emotional balance he was experiencing, and reported that he felt more energetic and invigorated. In addition, the restful sleep he had had during the last week was very effective in increasing his general feeling of energy.

After three months of treatment, there was an additional drop in Scott's blood pressure, which justified a certain reduction in his medications. His physician was deeply impressed with the success of the aromatherapy. He noticed the emotional changes in Scott, as manifested in his increased calmness and tranquillity as well as in the fact that he was slower to anger, and recommended that the treatment continue.

The treatment with oils brought about a significant improvement in Scott's mood and in his vigor and energy, and even after the conclusion of the series of massages, he continued to use the oil burner several times a day, "in order to feel good."

It is important to mention that when in-depth aromatherapy is performed as a solution to hypertension in a person who is being treated with medications, blood pressure must be tested regularly, preferably by a physician, since the oils (together with the massage and reflexology treatment techniques) and the medications operate simultaneously to reduce hypertension, and if the dosage of medications is not decreased, the client may suffer temporarily from low blood pressure. For this reason, it is important to work in conjunction with the client's physician.

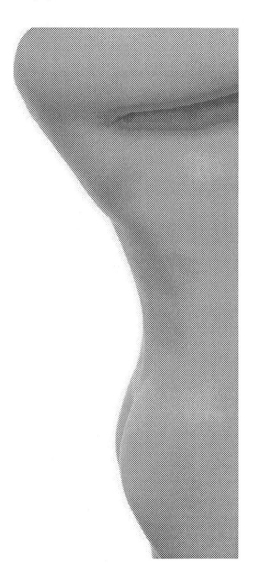 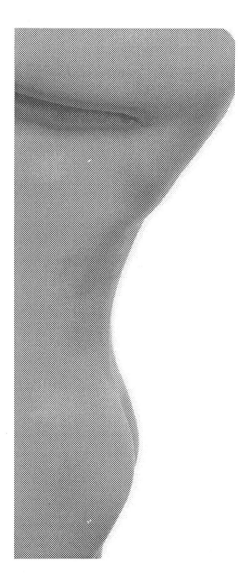

Hair loss

While Josh, a 34-year-old man, did not suffer from any particular health complaint, there was one problem that had begun to bother him over the last three years: increased hair loss. From the pre-treatment interview, it turned out that there was no hereditary hair loss in his family. Josh told me that after shampooing his hair, he would find a substantial amount of hair in his hands. In addition, when he combed his hair, he would see numerous hairs on the comb. But what frightened him the most was finding a lot of hairs on his pillow when he woke up in the morning. Josh had wavy, rather thick hair, which used to grow very densely and quickly, so that he would have his hair cut every two months. Now, he reckoned that his hair grew very slowly (besides the persistent hair loss problem) and looked thin.

Hair loss is a problem that afflicts many people nowadays. It can stem from genetic causes, such as a tendency toward baldness, from poor nutrition and from nutritional deficiencies, from various diseases, from contraceptive pills, and from anxiety, agitation, stress, and many other causes. In Josh's case, it seemed that the constant stress to which he was subjected, along with a weakening of the hair follicles for various reasons, were the causes of his hair loss. Aromatherapy for hair loss, especially when it is suspected that the problem is rooted in various emotional causes, is extremely effective. The treatment with oils should be carried out in conjunction with a scalp massage, which improves the blood flow and is very effective in halting the hair loss.

For preparing the blend, I used the carrier oil **jojoba**, which protects the skin against UV rays and is an excellent hair mask. I used 30 cc for preparing a blend in a 30-cc bottle. The essential oils I used were **rosemary** – one of the best-known oils for stopping hair loss and for treating the hair. **Rosemary** strengthens the hair, stimulates follicle growth, thereby accelerating the growth and regeneration of the hair, prevents hair loss, and is beneficial for the skin of the scalp. I dripped five drops of **rosemary** oil into the blend. The second oil I used was **lavender**. **Lavender** oil is known to accelerate growth after periods of hair loss. It strengthens the hair, and is very effective for people with thin hair. In addition, in Josh's case, **lavender** oil would calm him. I dripped five drops of this oil into the blend, and added five drops of **clary sage**, which, besides being a soothing oil, helps prevent hair loss, and is very good for the scalp, especially a greasy one.

Josh was to administer the treatment himself. I advised him to begin with a scalp massage with the oil blend three times a week for the first week. The massage had to be deep and long (about 15 minutes), using a generous amount of oil. After the massage, he was to cover his hair with a shower cap, leaving the blend on his hair for between a half-hour to two hours. Afterwards, he could wash his hair as usual, but preferably not with too much shampoo or conditioner (if they were not made from natural ingredients). During the second week, he was advised to use the hair mask twice, and during the third week, to use it once, and go on doing so for several months, or until the condition improved. In Josh's case, I also advised him to do relaxation exercises occasionally – preferably for a few minutes every day – and to calm down in the office, in order to reduce the amount of stress and pressure he was under.

Three weeks later, Josh already saw a change in the strength of his hair. His hair loss had also decreased a bit. Gradually, the hair loss ceased almost totally, and Josh noticed that the growth rate of his hair had returned to normal, as it had been in the past, before his problems had started. Now, four months after beginning the treatment, he hardly suffers from hair loss, and his hair has become as strong and thick as it was before. It is also healthier, shinier, and full of vitality. He is still using the oils in a scalp massage and a hair mask about once a week, and is very pleased with the results. Since he understood the possible link between hair loss and the high level of stress he suffered at work, he began to do relaxation exercises every day, and to calm down at work. Of course, these exercises give him a sensation of well being, tranquillity, and calmness, and fill him with energy, and it is certainly possible that they too contribute greatly to the significant reduction in hair loss.

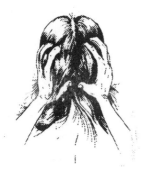

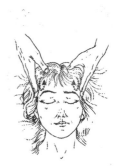

Problems in the respiratory system and problems common in the winter

When we treat problems in the respiratory system, especially chronic problems, we must pay attention to a number of factors:

The general condition of the immune system (this is also very significant in the treatment of infections and acute problems, especially if the person has a tendency to develop several respiratory tract infections every winter, and if he suffers, in addition, from fungal infections, eczema, and so on);

The person's emotional state (some diseases of the respiratory system, such as asthma, may have a psychosomatic aspect or may be exacerbated by situations of stress, pressure, depression, and so on). Emotional imbalance, depression, stress, periods of crisis, agitation, and so on greatly debilitate the immune system and interfere with its ability to "treat" the various viruses and toxins in the body naturally and effectively;

The third factor we have to examine is the existence of some kind of allergy that may cause various problems in the respiratory tract, such as asthma and hay fever. Many respiratory tract problems, such as infections, colds, acute bronchitis and acute sinusitis, occur during the winter. Some of the diseases that are caused by a bacterial infection occur after a slight chill, flu, or a slight viral disease that debilitates the immune system, thereby permitting bacteria to "settle" in the inflamed or infected area.

There is a broad range of oils that are suitable for treating problems of the respiratory tract and for treating winter diseases. Some of them have a rather high level of toxicity, and it is therefore necessary to substitute milder oils when we want to treat children, elderly people, or people with a low level of vitality (weak or sickly people).

Among the most common oils for treating respiratory tract infections and similar problems that arise during the winter are the following essential oils:

Eucalyptus oil is one of the best-known oils for treating respiratory problems and diseases. This oil is anti-inflammatory for the respiratory tract and antiviral (it helps the immune system attack viruses in the respiratory tract). It is good for treating asthma, chronic bronchitis and acute bronchitis, for congestion in the respiratory tract, and for treating throat infections, colds and chills. The oil is an expectorant, is good for treating sinusitis and coughs, relaxes spasms in the respiratory tract, and also serves as a treatment for flu and pneumonia (in conjunction with medical treatment).

It must be remembered that **eucalyptus** oil is not suitable for treating infants, and **niaouli** oil can be used instead.

Lemon oil reinforces the immune system and expedites the production of leukocytes (white blood cells that fight infection). It is effective in treating bronchitis (especially together with **bergamot** oil), throat infections and various respiratory tract infections (since it is a very powerful antibacterial oil), colds and chills, runny noses and sinusitis.

Peppermint oil is also very common in the treatment of respiratory tract problems. This oil opens the respiratory tract and disinfects it. It is an expectorant and is antispasmodic for the respiratory tract. It is suitable for treating asthma, chronic bronchitis, congestion in the respiratory tract, headaches resulting from diseases of the respiratory tract, colds, chills, and sinusitis.

Basil oil helps when there is phlegm. It is an expectorant, and helps treat flu and barking coughs.

Frankincense oil is very effective in the treatment of asthma, bronchitis, congestion in the respiratory tract, throat and respiratory tract infections, in soothing conditions of hyperventilation and shortness of breath, and in treating sinusitis and coughs. In addition, it is an effective expectorant.

Chamomile oil, too, is very effective in the treatment of a range of winter and respiratory tract diseases. It reinforces the immune system, promotes the production of leukocytes, is effective in the treatment of infections of the respiratory tract, and prevents the development of secondary infections. It is effective in the treatment of flu, bronchitis (especially if combined with **niaouli**), congestion in the respiratory tract, colds and chills, and runny noses and flu. Moreover, it is important to note its excellent work on the mental level.

Cinnamon oil also reinforces the immune system, and is good for treating respiratory tract infections and for preventing recurring infections, for treating colds and chills, breathing difficulties and flu, and it generally reinforces the respiratory system. It must not be used during pregnancy, and is not suitable for use with infants and small children. Moreover, it should not be used on the face.

Lavender oil is also effective in treating an array of respiratory tract problems. It reinforces the immune system, promotes the production of leukocytes, helps in cases of congestion and phlegm, is suitable for treating sinusitis, chills and colds, soothes the respiratory tract, and is very good used in combination with **niaouli**. Of course, its properties that treat various emotional states effectively should also be taken into account.

Benzoin oil reinforces the respiratory system, helps in conditions of congestion in the respiratory tract, asthma, bronchitis, infections of the respiratory tract, and throat infections, treats colds and chills (especially following exposure to cold and damp). It is suitable for all conditions of congestion and phlegm, cleans out the respiratory tract, and expands respiration. It can be used for coughs and for rehabilitating and strengthening the mucus membranes of the respiratory tract.

Angelica oil is suitable for treating colds and chills, congestion and phlegm, flu, bronchitis, congestion in the respiratory tract, sinusitis, lung congestion (only when treatment is administered by an experienced and professional aromatherapist together with medical treatment) and flu. It must not be used during pregnancy.

Cedarwood oil has the unusual property of rehabilitating and strengthening the mucus membranes of the respiratory system and generally treating mucus membranes. Moreover, it helps in conditions of congestion and phlegm, coughs, congestion in the respiratory tract, and bronchitis.

Sandalwood oil is an antispasmodic oil for the respiratory system, and for this reason is often used in the treatment of asthma. It is suitable for treating bronchitis, for infections of the respiratory tract and sore throats, for treating hoarseness and coughs, and is also an expectorant. In addition, it has relaxing properties and is emotionalyl strengthening.

Red thyme and **sweet thyme** oils are also considered extremely effective oils in the treatment of a range of respiratory tract diseases. Although both of them are effective, I mainly recommend using **sweet thyme**, because of its low level of toxicity, while **red thyme** has a higher level of toxicity, and must not be used with children and infants.

Sweet thyme oil reinforces the immune system, promotes the production of leukocytes, is antispasmodic for the respiratory system, and is effective in the treatment of asthma, bronchitis, sore throats, and tonsillitis (a drop of it can be placed on a cotton bud and then applied to the infectious spots on the tonsils; it is advisable for someone with good eyes and a steady hand to administer the treatment gently). It is an expectorant and helps in the treatment of congestion and phlegm, sinusitis, pneumonia (along with medical treatment), coughs and flu.

Tea tree oil also reinforces the immune system and helps in conditions of congestion and phlegm. It disinfects the respiratory tract, is antibacterial, treats runny noses, sinusitis, throat infections and bacterial conditions, and congestion in the respiratory tract.

Petitgrain oil reinforces the immune system and is suitable for the treatment of sinusitis. It also has emotionally soothing and encouraging properties.

Cypress oil is antispasmodic for the respiratory system, is suitable for the treatment of bronchitis and conditions of congestion in the respiratory system, soothes the nerves of the respiratory system, is good for treating spastic coughs and flu, and for rehabilitating and strengthening the mucus membranes of the respiratory system.

Niaouli oil is also suitable for treating flu, lung problems (in conjunction with appropriate medical treatment), throat infections and respiratory tract infections, congestion in the respiratory tract, asthma and bronchitis.

Camphor oil is suitable for treating infections in the respiratory system, colds and chills, but its use is not recommended because of its high level of toxicity.

Fennel oil is superb for soothing coughs and for treating hoarseness. It is also considered to be a good expectorant, but it is important to remember that it must not be used on children, pregnant women, and epileptics.

Clary sage oil is suitable for the treatment of asthma and shortness of breath (especially when these conditions are accompanied by fear or stem from mental stress). It is antispasmodic for the windpipe, and has excellent properties for treating emotional states of fear, tension, and depression. It must not be used during pregnancy or in conjunction with alcohol.

Pine oil is also good for a range of respiratory tract problems and for treating chronic and acute bronchitis, as is **myrtle** oil, which is recommended for the treatment of children. It is an antiseptic and expectorant oil that is suitable for the treatment of flu, bronchitis, and colds. **Rosemary** oil is also suitable for the treatment of flu. It also helps relieve congestion in the respiratory tract, and is suitable for treating asthma and sinusitis. **Myrrh** oil, which is known to dry excess phlegm and to be an expectorant, is used in the treatment of lung diseases (of course, in conjunction with medical treatment), for rehabilitation of the mucus membranes of the respiratory tract, and in the treatment of hoarseness, sore throats, congestion in the respiratory tract, and chronic bronchitis.

There are many other oils that are used for treating various problems of the respiratory tract, but the ones mentioned above are the best known and are used for treating a very broad range of problems.

In general, the primary method for treating respiratory tract problems with essential oils is, of course, inhalation. In the chapter on methods of treatment, there are instructions for preparing an inhalation. By inhaling steam during an inhalation, the essential oils reach the respiratory tract and affect it, but it must be remembered that **this type of treatment is not suitable for asthma sufferers**.

Another excellent way of treating respiratory tract infections, and especially viral and bacterial diseases, is via an oil burner. As a rule, when someone in the household gets a cold, flu, or any other disease that may be contagious and spread germs or viruses, it is highly recommended to light an oil burner containing suitable oils (antibacterial, antiviral, and disinfectant oils) in order to prevent the spread of the disease to other members of the household. In cases in which there are pains or congestion in the face or chest region because of a respiratory tract disease, a cough, or an infection, it is a good idea to perform a pleasant, warming local massage of the area.

For treating respiratory tract infections in children and infants during the winter, it is advisable to use one of the following oils, which are suitable for children and infants because of their low level of toxicity: **myrtle**, **lavender**, **niaouli**, **frankincense**, and **chamomile**.

Since these oils encompass most of the respiratory tract problems, there is no need to use other oils that can harm infants and small children.

Hay fever

Mike, a 45-year-old businessman, came into the clinic, and it didn't take a genius to guess what was bothering him. His eyes were watering and looked red and inflamed, he announced his entrance with sneezes, and he held a crushed Kleenex in his hand. During those late spring and early summer days, when the air was filled with pollen, it was easy to guess that Mike was suffering from hay fever. Every time spring turned into summer, it was the same story. Mike, a well-built, generally healthy man who devoted a lot of time to himself, to his personal grooming and to the development of body and mind, found himself laid low over and over again by the tiresome signs and symptoms that characterize this allergy.

In addition, because of the inflamed condition of his respiratory system during the attack of hay fever, Mike also suffered from annoying headaches.

Hay fever is a disease that resembles asthma by nature, except that in this disease, the symptoms are expressed in the eyes, the nose, and the throat, and not in the lungs or chest cavity, as with asthma sufferers. As with asthma, here, too, the allergic reaction is caused by airborne substances. These substances are generally pollen, tiny fragments of animal fur (especially cats), dust, and various chemical substances. The substance that triggers the allergy causes the secretion of a chemical called histamine in the person's body, and this produces an inflammation and the secretion of liquids in the eyelids, in the external layer of the eyes, and in the nasal cavities.

The disease is very widespread in the US and Western Europe.

The reason for the disease is not known. Those same allergic substances that cause an allergic reaction in one person do not cause a similar reaction in another person, and the hypotheses regarding the reason for the disease point mainly at the genetic factor, since there are families in which there is a history of hay fever. However, new research tends to suppose that the causes of the disease are actually environmental and climatic.

Hay fever is more common in people under 40, people who suffer from other allergies, people who suffer from asthma or eczema, and people in whose families there are others who suffer from some kind of allergy.

Hay fever is characterized by the appearance of redness, burning, itching and watering in the eyes, repetitive sneezing, and a clear liquid runny nose. In addition to these symptoms, some people also experience a burning or dryness in the throat, wheezing, and itchy skin. Sometimes, the symptoms appear in the form of an attack of watering eyes and sneezing that continues for a quarter to a half-hour, and gradually dies down.

There are various types of hay fever, and the problem can be permanent or seasonal. The most common seasons for suffering from seasonal hay fever are spring and summer, when plants bloom and emit their pollen.

This disease is not dangerous, but it can be very annoying, and sometimes, in extreme cases, is liable to disrupt the person's everyday functioning and interfere with his normal life. The treatments dispensed by physicians include various antihistamines, and, in more serious cases, steroids, which have many side effects and do not treat the root of the problem, but rather only the symptoms. In order to treat the root of the problem, the cause must be identified, and then the sensitivity must be neutralized. This treatment is performed by an allergy specialist, and can go on for a long time.

I explained to Mike that the most effective treatment for preventing the disease itself was treatment that focused on discovering the allergic causes and neutralizing his body's sensitivity to these causes. However, it turned out that Mike had known about this treatment for a long time, and had even considered trying it. He was more interested in a relieving and supportive treatment that would help him get through the difficult period of the disease more smoothly and easily.

As a relieving and supportive treatment, inhalation of essential oils can be very effective. It can relieve the attacks, soothe them, support the health of the organs that are suffering from the allergy, and generally fortify the person who is suffering, in order to help him cope with the annoying duration of the hay fever attack.

The oils that are suitable for use in an inhalation are **myrtle**, which is very suitable for use in various respiratory problems, and is also suitable for use in children because of its mildness; **pine**, which is known to relieve respiratory problems; **eucalyptus**, which is a bit strong and not recommended for use in children, but is very effective in almost all respiratory tract problems, relieves congestion, is effective for treating asthma and inflammatory conditions in the respiratory system, and is an expectorant; **cajeput**, which is antispasmodic, effective in treating a range of respiratory tract problems and infections, helps in cases of irregular breathing, and purifies the system; **tea tree**, which disinfects the system, helps congestion and diseases in the respiratory tract, and relieves phlegm and runny noses; **lemon**, which is suitable for treating a broad range of respiratory tract problems and infections, and for runny noses; **thyme**, which is also suitable for a broad range of respiratory tract problems, antispasmodic, effective as a treatment for asthma, relieves sore throats, and is an expectorant; **marigold**, which soothes the system and is antispasmodic; **petitgrain**, which is also soothing and antispasmodic and relates to the emotional side of the allergic problem; and **peppermint**, which is antispasmodic for the respiratory system, serves as a treatment for asthma, disinfects the system, and can relieve congestion in the respiratory system as well as the headaches that are caused by congestion in the respiratory tract.

Eucalyptus, **thyme**, **pine**, and **peppermint** oils help in the treatment of allergic conditions, and this is the reason for their great effectiveness in the treatment of hay fever. Out of all those oils, it is advisable to choose two, and to drip two to four drops of each of them into the inhalation appliance. If you don't have an inhalation appliance that is suitable for use with oils, the oils can be dripped into a regular steam appliance, in the special place for this purpose, or into the bowl of water – drip the oils into a wide bowl containing a liter of hot (not boiling) steaming water. The person must bend his head over the bowl – with a towel covering his head in order to ensure that the steam reaches his face – and inhale the fragrant steam for a few minutes.

For Mike, I prepared a blend from **pine** and **peppermint**, which would also help relieve the headaches that resulted from the congestion in his nose and respiratory tract. I recommended that he do the inhalation every day for a few minutes in order to relieve the symptoms of the disease, release the congestion in his nose, and ease his breathing.

Moreover, I prepared a chest massage blend for him, in which I used **sunflower** oil as a carrier oil, into which I dripped equal quantities of **peppermint** and **pine**. In principle, in order to prepare a blend for a single massage, you can take one tablespoon of **sunflower** oil, and drip one of the oils used in the inhalation, or one of the oils that is suitable for treating hay fever. The massage should be performed with slow, gentle, circular movements, although the chest can also be rubbed gently.

In order to relieve the burning sensation Mike felt in his throat, I suggested that he drip one drop of **tea tree** oil and one drop of **lemon** oil into a cup of lukewarm water, and gargle carefully, avoiding swallowing the liquid. The gargle liquid disinfects the throat very effectively, is important in preventing the spread of viruses or bacteria over the inflamed and debilitated system, and greatly relieves the burning in the throat.

Mike followed my instructions meticulously. The inhalation improved the state of his blocked, congested, dripping nose, and about three hours later, he still felt enormous relief in his breathing – a kind of cleanliness and openness in his congested respiratory tract. The state of burning and watering eyes also improved a bit after the inhalation. Mike used the inhalation every day for the two weeks during which he suffered from sneezing attacks, an inflamed throat, a runny nose and watering eyes, and felt significant relief during the day. In general, he began his day with the inhalation in order to make the rest of the day easier, but sometimes, when he felt a lot of congestion during the night, and this bothered him and interfered with his sleep, he did it again at night, and this helped him get through the night better.

Mike performed the massage once a day, by himself, and found that this greatly relieved his breathing, and soothed his inflamed respiratory tract. The gargle mixture did not effect a substantial change in the burning sensation in his throat for the first two days he used it, but on the third day, he began to feel a relief in the burning, which gradually increased.

Mike felt that this time, his hay fever had been much easier and more comfortable. The tiresome symptoms bothered him less, and he got through the two weeks (which were usually torture for him, and totally disruptive for his daily routine) much more easily.

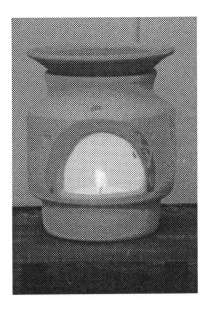

Asthma

Andy, a man of about 42, came for aromatherapy because of the asthma from which he had been suffering for many years.

Asthma (spastic bronchitis) is a very common disease. About 10% of children and about 5% of adults suffer from it. In some of the cases, there is a familial tendency. Asthma is one of the most common childhood diseases. In 90% of cases, it appears by age four (if it has not appeared by then, the chances of it appearing later are small).

Andy could not remember when his asthma started, but he recalled himself as a slightly sickly child, weak and asthmatic. In fact, since he could remember, he had suffered from asthma. Between ages five and eight, the disease was especially severe, and was accompanied by very powerful attacks of shortness of breath. He had been treated with Ventolin for many years, and now, although his attacks were weaker and less frequent, he always ensured that he had a Ventolin inhaler with him wherever he went. During his military service, the asthma decreased to a great extent, and the attacks became rare and milder – but nevertheless bothersome when they did occur. About five years before coming to see me, the intensity and frequency of Andy's attacks increased, and he was worried about this. His shortness of breath would occur mainly in the morning, and he reckoned that during periods of stress and tension, the attacks were far more frequent.

I have divided the treatment of asthma with essential oils into two conditions:
1. Treatment of asthma during an attack. (It is important to remember that in Andy's case, the attacks were not extreme, nor did they reach a stage of exceptional or suffocating shortness of breath, so they could be treated with aromatherapy.) *Under no circumstances* must a powerful asthma attack (which does not subside even after inhaling Ventolin) be treated with essential oils. The person must get medical treatment.

Even in the case of an attack that is not extreme, if the oils do not help within a few minutes, *an inhaler or a medication prescribed by a physician must be used!* Asthma attacks can escalate very fast and become dangerous, so chances must not be taken in such cases!
2. A fixed daily treatment in order to improve the general feeling and to "open" Andy's "blocked" nose, a treatment that gradually gave him significant relief and caused a gradual decrease in the frequency and intensity of the attacks.

In order to calm the attack, I suggested that Andy choose one of the following oils: **peppermint, myrtle, frankincense, eucalyptus, spearmint,** or **pine**. When he felt the onset of shortness of breath, he was to drip two drops of one of the oils onto a Kleenex and inhale its vapor. I asked him to use each oil for two days until he found the one that gave him the greatest relief from shortness of breath.

Moreover, I prepared a blend for an oil burner, containing (in a 10-cc bottle) 15 drops of **eucalyptus** oil, 25 drops of **myrtle** oil, and 15 drops of **frankincense** oil, which is very helpful in situations of stress as well, since it soothes and heals (this would help Andy during attacks of shortness of breath brought on by tension).

Andy tried the oils for calming his asthma attacks and found that **frankincense** oil helped him regulate his breathing and calm down within a short time. Moreover, he mentioned that he really liked its fragrance, so he chose this oil to carry with him.

Since **frankincense** oil helped calm the asthma attacks effectively, albeit more slowly than inhaling Ventolin, Andy thought that he would no longer take his Ventolin inhaler with him, and just take the bottle of essential oil. I explained to him that he should not take unnecessary risks. If the **frankincense** oil helped him so much, he should carry it with him all the time – along with his Ventolin inhaler. As long as the **frankincense** oil helped soothe his attacks, he should use it, but if for some reason a situation should occur in which it did not help, his Ventolin inhaler should be at hand.

Andy used the oil burner every day, sometimes several times a day – at work as well. He told me that the oil vapors that filled the small office gave him a feeling of well being and enabled him to breathe more easily, and every now and then he felt his nose "open" up as well. In addition, he mentioned that the vapors gave the office a pleasant atmosphere, calmed him, and helped him feel less pressured. When he felt as if his nose was blocked to the point that he could neither smell nor breathe through it, he would inhale the drops of **frankincense** oil he had dripped onto a Kleenex, and often felt significant relief in the opening of his respiratory passages.

During the year, Andy made sure to eat properly and to exercise – swimming – and even lost 14 pounds. The weight loss and the physical activity contributed greatly to calming his asthma attacks down, but he still used the oil burner occasionally when he felt the need, or inhaled the **frankincense** from the Kleenex when he felt shortness of breath.

Sinusitis

Allie, a 22-year-old first-year naturology student, requested an effective treatment for relieving the sinusitis pains from which she had been suffering. Since she was studying naturology, a subject that is connected to essential oils, among other things, she wanted to test the efficacy of the essential oil treatment in cases of acute infections, such as sinusitis. For a few days, Allie had been suffering from severe pain in her face and forehead, from headaches, and from congestion and a runny nose.

When treating sinusitis, we have a choice of many treatment options with essential oils. We try to reinforce the client's immune system in general, and to match the choice of oils to his specific physical or mental needs. Among the essential oils that are recommended for the treatment of sinusitis is **eucalyptus** oil, which is also antiviral, stimulating, invigorating, and an expectorant; **angelica** oil, which is a powerful disinfectant and bactericide, as well as being warming and soothing. Like **eucalyptus**, it is also suitable for treating a broad range of respiratory tract problems; **tea tree** oil, a powerful disinfectant, antiviral and antibacterial, which reinforces the immune system, helps in conditions of congestion and phlegm, disinfects the respiratory tract, and is suitable for treating sinusitis and congestion in the respiratory tract; **niaouli** oil, which is also antibacterial and is especially suitable for treating sinusitis in children; **cajeput** oil, which is suitable for treating a broad range of respiratory tract problems, especially sinusitis that occurs after a cold; it, too, is antiviral and stimulating; **lemon** oil, with its powerful antibacterial properties that help treat a broad range of viral problems in the respiratory tract and help reinforce the immune system; **lavender** oil, which, besides its wonderful properties for relieving tension and mental stress – which may jeopardize recovery – also reinforces the immune system. **Sweet thyme** oil also reinforces the immune system, promotes leukocyte production, is antispasmodic in the respiratory system, and is effective for treating sinusitis. It is also an expectorant and helps treat conditions of congestion and phlegm. Because of its relatively low level of toxicity, it is preferable to **red thyme**. **Petitgrain** oil is antiviral, reinforces the immune system, and has soothing and encouraging emotional properties that can help us in treating the client's emotional condition. **Rosemary** oil, too, which helps congestion in the respiratory tract, is suitable for treating sinusitis.

As in any aromatic treatment, I inquired about Allie's general state of physical and emotional health. Her state of health was completely normal, and she did not have any physical problems, even though she suffered from colds, flu, and various respiratory infections several times each winter. This meant that her immune system had to be reinforced. From the emotional point of view, she attested to being a calm person, "always" in a good mood. Lately, however, because of her work and studies, her crowded days, her demanding study schedule, deadlines for handing in papers, and hard work, she often found herself suffering from stress and tension, unable to calm down.

The essential oils I chose for Allie's treatment were **angelica** and **lavender**. The latter reinforces the immune system and calms and releases tension. It is also very effective when used in an inhalation. The treatment that is recommended for sinusitis is, of course, inhalation, because the oil vapors reach the respiratory tract directly. The inhalation can be done using a bowl containing a liter of hot (not boiling), steaming water containing five drops of the blend. The person's head must be covered with a towel and held over the bowl, creating a kind of "tent" effect that prevents the vapors from escaping. It is also possible to drip several drops of the essential oil into a steam appliance or into an inhalation appliance, but it is important to consult the manufacturer's directions as to whether essential oils can be dripped into it. There are also special inhalation appliances that are particularly suitable for aromatherapy treatments.

In addition, I prepared a blend of essential oils for a facial massage in order to relieve congestion and the unpleasant feeling around Allie's nose and eyes. I prepared the blend from 10 cc of **almond** oil, into which I dripped two drops of **angelica** oil and three drops of **lavender** oil. I asked Allie to perform the massage gently, concentrating on the forehead and nose areas, which were congested, and avoiding contact with the eyes (this is important when massaging the face!).

Allie performed the inhalation every day, sometimes even twice a day, and massaged her face morning and evening, before going to bed, in order to facilitate sleep. She reported a great improvement in her condition. Her illness was shorter than usual and much less severe, and within a few days, Allie was her old self again, refreshed and strengthened.

Acute bronchitis and chronic bronchitis

Chronic bronchitis is the result of constant damage of the mucus membrane of the respiratory tract – especially the alveoli – by cigarettes. Chronic bronchitis is defined as follows: when there are three consecutive months of productive coughing (that is, coughing in which a greeny-yellow phlegm is produced) for two years (three consecutive months each time). In principle, the disease is mainly caused by a chronic irritation of the mucus membranes of the respiratory tract by foreign substances, smoke among them, resulting in over-secretion by the mucus membranes of the respiratory tract, disruption of the action of the cilia (hairs) of the respiratory tract, disruption of the concentration of the secretions from the respiratory tract, and disruption of the functioning of the cells responsible for fighting and eliminating bacteria and viruses from the respiratory tract.

In the first stages of the disease, there is usually a cough with expectoration (a productive cough), mainly in winter and mainly in the morning. The expectoration is whitish, but later becomes murky and pus-like, and appears during most of the hours of the day. As the disease progresses, it also appears during most months of the year. Moreover, the amounts of expectoration gradually increase. The person coughs for longer periods and more frequently. At the end of each attack of coughing, wheezing occurs as a result of the narrowing of the vocal cords. When, in addition, there is a severe infection (bacterial or viral) in the respiratory tract, the situation worsens, sometimes even drastically.

When we treat chronic bronchitis, it is important first and foremost to eliminate the factor that led to the development of the chronic infection of the vocal cords (usually smoking). By so doing, especially in the first stages of the disease, it is possible to halt the inflammatory process and effect a recovery of the respiratory tract. If the process continues despite the elimination of the causing factor, and especially if there is evidence of a bacterial infection, antibiotic treatment is recommended, in accordance with expectoration cultures and the sensitivity of the bacteria. In people with a severe infection, who suffer from recurring attacks of bacterial infections during certain periods (particularly the winter), the physician sometimes prescribes preventive antibiotic treatment for the duration of the problematic period. The physician sometimes prescribes expectorant medications for a client with chronic bronchitis, medications that decrease the viscosity of the sputum, and enable it to be eliminated more effectively, and medications that widen the vocal cords for clients suffering from a narrowing of the vocal cords.

Additional reasons – besides smoking – that can cause chronic bronchitis are exposure to dust, pollen, particles of animal fur, and various chemical factors, and exposure to them should be avoided as much as possible.

For people who suffer from chronic bronchitis, it is important and advisable to do aerobic exercises in order to help the respiratory system. Swimming, gym workouts, and aerobics can improve their condition. It is vital to quit smoking and to treat the disease, since chronic bronchitis causes damage to the lungs, and can cause complications and act as a catalyst in the development of other diseases, such as pulmonary hypertension, emphysema (an extremely serious lung disease), inadequate functioning of the right side of the heart, and pneumonia.

Acute bronchitis (a severe inflammation of the vocal cords), as opposed to chronic bronchitis, is not caused by smoking, but rather by an infection of the respiratory tract. After a cold or a jaw infection, infection-causing germs can spread downward and penetrate the vocal cords. The disease is expressed in a fever, an irritating cough that produces a yellowish expectoration, and a feeling of irritation in the chest (which tends to continue for a few days after the infection disappears), shortness of breath, and sometimes chest pains that are more severe when coughing, nausea, and appetite loss. In children and infants, restlessness can be observed during the incubation period of the disease. In cases of an isolated attack, when the person does not smoke and the bronchitis attacks are rare (once every few years), the disease is not dangerous, and can be treated at home (a successful treatment will cause the fever to go down). In the case of a very high fever, it is important to undergo medical tests. However, when the person smokes, the attacks of bronchitis are liable to recur over and over again, and then it is necessary to consult with a physician.

In cases of both chronic bronchitis and acute bronchitis, it is important to see that, in addition to treatments, the person drinks large amounts of fluids, especially fruit juices and juices that contain a large quantity of vitamin C, herbal tea, and water, in order to soften the respiratory secretions and enable the sputum to be expectorated. It is also important to do breathing exercises in order to aerate every part of the lung, especially the parts that are blocked by sputum, particularly in the case of chronic bronchitis. When infants or elderly people suffer from this disease, they must immediately undergo medical treatment in order to avoid the development of additional problematic conditions in the respiratory tract.

In order to treat chronic and acute bronchitis, we use expectorant oils – oils that help treat the congestion in the respiratory system – antiviral and antibacterial oils, anti-inflammatory oils, oils that reinforce the immune and the respiratory systems, and, if the person has a history of allergies, we include oils that treat allergies (such as **chamomile**) in the blend.

Among the essential oils that are suitable for treating bronchitis are the following: **eucalyptus** oil, which is anti-inflammatory for the respiratory system, antiviral, an expectorant, and suitable for treating congestion in the respiratory system, very effective in treating chronic and severe bronchitis; **lemon** oil, which is important in the treatment of bronchitis because it reinforces the immune system and catalyzes the production of leukocytes. It is effective in the treatment of bronchitis especially in conjunction with **bergamot** oil, and it is also a very powerful antibacterial oil; **basil** oil, which is suitable for treating chronic and acute bronchitis because it helps with phlegm congestion, it is an expectorant, and it is effective in relieving coughs; **oregano** oil, which is also suitable for treating bronchitis, and has good disinfectant properties.

Peppermint oil opens the respiratory system and disinfects it. It is an expectorant and helps treat congestion in the respiratory system. It is especially suitable for treating chronic bronchitis. **Frankincense** oil is also very effective in the treatment of bronchitis and congestion in the respiratory system. It is an expectorant and helps relieve coughs.

Chamomile oil reinforces the immune system, is effective in the treatment of respiratory tract infections, and prevents the development of secondary infections. It helps treat congestion in the respiratory system, and in the treatment of bronchitis, it should be combined with **niaouli** oil in the blend. These two oils are wonderful for treating acute bronchitis in children and infants, but, of course, in these cases, a physician must be consulted.

Lavender oil is also effective in the treatment of a range of respiratory tract problems, reinforces the immune system, promotes leukocyte production, and, with **niaouli** oil, helps treat congestion. **Niaouli** oil is also suitable for treating bronchitis and congestion in the respiratory tract, as is **myrtle** oil, which is an antiseptic and expectorant oil, and is effective in the treatment of bronchitis.

Remember that the five last oils – **lavender, chamomile, niaouli, myrtle,** and **frankincense** – are the oils with which we treat children and infants.

Benzoin oil reinforces the respiratory system, helps treat congestion in the respiratory tract, is suitable for treating respiratory tract and throat infections, as well as phlegm congestion, and is very effective in the treatment of bronchitis because it cleans the respiratory tract and "broadens" the breathing, rehabilitates and strengthens the mucus membranes in the respiratory tract, and is very effective in the treatment of coughs.

Tea tree oil is important in the treatment of bronchitis because of its properties of reinforcing the immune system, disinfecting the respiratory system, and helping treat phlegm congestion in the respiratory system. In addition, it is a very powerful antibacterial oil.

Cypress oil soothes the nerves of the respiratory system, and because it is antispasmodic, it is suitable for treating spastic coughs. The oil also helps relieve congestion in the respiratory tract, and is very suitable for the treatment of chronic bronchitis since it contributes to the rehabilitation and strengthening of the mucus membranes of the respiratory system. **Cedarwood** oil, too, contains the important property of rehabilitating and strengthening the mucus membranes of the respiratory system and is important for the general treatment of the mucus membranes. For this reason, it helps and is important in the treatment of mainly chronic bronchitis. In addition, it also helps treat phlegm congestion and congestion in the respiratory system and relieves coughs, which makes it an excellent oil with which to treat the problem. **Angelica** oil is also suitable for treating bronchitis because it relieves phlegm congestion and congestion in the respiratory tract. **Sweet thyme** oil, which reinforces the immune system and promotes leukocyte production, is also antispasmodic for the respiratory system and effective in the treatment of phlegm congestion. It is an expectorant and is suitable for treating coughs. **Sandalwood** oil is an expectorant and antispasmodic oil for the respiratory system, and it too is suitable for treating bronchitis and respiratory tract infections. It helps relieve hoarseness and coughs. **Myrrh** oil, which dries up excessive phlegm and is an expectorant, is also suitable for treating mainly chronic bronchitis, and it also helps rehabilitate the mucus membranes of the respiratory system and treat hoarseness and congestion in the respiratory tract.

In addition, **pine** oil is suitable for treating chronic and acute bronchitis, as are **rosemary** and **laurel** oil.

Out of this wide range of oils that can treat bronchitis, it is important to find the oils that are suitable for the person's general condition, and if there are additional physical problems or sensitivities, these must be taken into account when preparing the blend of essential oils.

In the treatment of chronic bronchitis, it is a good idea to include oils for reinforcing the immune system in the blend in order to lower the level of contagion by various viral and bacterial diseases. The strengthening of the immune system will enable it to cope with the germs. Moreover, oils for increasing concentration and for relaxation can also be added to the blend.

The preferred oils for treatment are **rosemary**, which, besides being excellent for treating bronchitis, also stimulates and clarifies thought and increases concentration; **basil**, which, besides being suitable for treating chronic bronchitis and phlegm congestion, for relieving coughs and expectoration, also stimulates and clarifies thought; **frankincense**, which, besides being very effective in treating congestion in the respiratory tract, relieving coughs, expectorating, and effective in treating bronchitis, also has a calming action; and **lavender**, which, besides being suitable for treating bronchitis, also reinforces the immune system effectively, and is wonderfully soothing. Since we are treating this problem in three stages, we will also add **eucalyptus** oil, which is an extraordinarily effective oil for treating bronchitis, and it is also antiviral and antibacterial.

The first stage of the treatment is very simple, but is very important and must be performed meticulously. You must tell the client to drink a lot of fluids during the day in order to soften the secretions from the respiratory tract and to facilitate their expectoration. By drinking a lot, he will clean his body and help the essential oils work more easily. The client should drink mainly herbal tea such as chamomile, which is soothing, or peppermint, which is slightly stimulating and may increase his level of concentration, as well as being beneficial for the respiratory system. Moreover, he should drink natural juices, especially those that contain a high level of vitamin C (it is a good idea to take one or two vitamin C tablets a day in order to reinforce the ability of the immune system to cope with the smoking damage that the client has suffered from for years). The natural juices should be diluted with water in order to ensure that they are not too thick, thereby making expectoration difficult.

The second stage is the daily massage of the chest and back. I prepared the massage blend from 20 cc of **grapeseed** oil in which I dripped five drops of **wheatgerm** oil, three drops of **eucalyptus** oil, and two drops of **basil** oil. The massage must be performed once a day for 20 minutes, preferably in the morning, when the state of the bronchitis is more severe, and the coughing and phlegm are particularly disturbing. Over time, as the annoying symptoms decrease, the frequency of the massage can be reduced to alternate days. The chest massage should be performed with warming, circular movements that open the chest, from the center outward.

The third stage is filling the room with essential oil vapors from an oil burner. As a blend for the burner, I chose **frankincense, rosemary,** and **lavender** oils – four drops of each. Moreover, one of the essential oils can be replaced each time with **eucalyptus** or **basil** in order to have a more varied blend.

The use of the oil burner is recommended for the workplace as well, since the blend contains oils that are soothing during times of pressure at work, and improve the powers of concentration. At times when there are people who are ill with viral or bacterial infections at home or at work, it is a good idea to substitute **eucalyptus** oil for one of the oils, because it is very effective in disinfecting the room and killing germs.

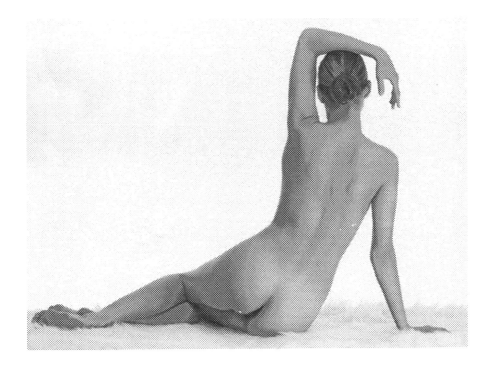

Colds

A friend of mine, Denise, suffered from colds. Very quickly, her nose would begin to drip, her throat would burn and ache, and she would cough and get a blocked nose and generally feel bad. In order to ease her symptoms, she asked me for essential oils that would help her feel better.

Colds are caused by viruses, and, of course, are not dangerous to people who are usually healthy; however, they are certainly not pleasant, either. (When people with immune system diseases, weak elderly people, seriously ill people or weak and sensitive infants have colds, it is important to get medical treatment.) In general, the symptoms are a runny nose, a blocked nose, coughing, a sore and irritated throat, and sometimes a headache because of the congestion in the respiratory tract. With colds, the person's temperature is not likely to rise more than one degree above normal (as opposed to flu, in which the temperature can rise to above 100 degrees Fahrenheit).

I first suggested to Denise that she drink a lot of herbal tea. Drinking a lot of mainly warm beverages softens the respiratory tract secretions and helps the immune system in its fight against germs. Herbal tea, especially infusions, has a lot of added value because of the wonderful action of medicinal herbs. In cases of colds, tea made from black danewort, ginger, melissa, sage, angelica, rosemary, hyssop, nettle, eucalyptus, and thyme can bring substantial relief, and tea made from basil can be very effective in treating coughs.

Moreover, it is highly recommended that a person with a cold eat raw onion because of its excellent antibiotic properties, or put a peeled clove of garlic in his mouth, hold it in the hollow of his cheeks, next to the back teeth, and move it from one side of his mouth to the other for a few minutes. If possible, he should chew the garlic. Another method that is recommended for the intrepid is to drip one drop of freshly squeezed lemon juice into each nostril, bending the head backward. Of course, this doesn't feel great, but, because of the lemon's acidity, the mucus membranes shrink, thus reducing the secretion of runny mucus. Taking vitamin C several times a day also affords significant relief, and strengthens and vitalizes the immune system so that it can cope with "invaders" successfully. An echinacea and propolis preparation, which can be purchased at drugstores, can be excellent for treating or even preventing colds when it is taken regularly on a daily basis during the winter in order to strengthen the immune system and preempt infection.

Besides these methods of treatment, I suggested that Denise take a hot shower. Over and above the relief provided by freshening up, the hot water softens the respiratory tract secretions, and the steam helps open the blocked nose, giving a good feeling of "open" breathing. After the shower, it is easier to expel the mucus secretions when blowing the nose, and the overall feeling improves.

After the shower, I told Denise to drip a few drops of some of the following essential oils onto a Kleenex: **eucalyptus**, **lavender**, **sandalwood**, **tea tree**, **chamomile**, **cinnamon**, **lemon**, **niaouli**, **peppermint**, **oregano**, **basil**, **pine**, **myrtle**, **frankincense**, **laurel** or **rosemary**. When children have colds, we drip a drop or two of **niaouli**, **myrtle** or **frankincense** oil onto a Kleenex. Because of their low level of toxicity, they are suitable for treating children. Moreover, it is a good idea to drip a few drops of the chosen oil onto the pillow, so that the vapors can be inhaled during sleep. **Peppermint** oil is not recommended for this purpose, since it can cause bad dreams.

Denise chose to drip a few drops of **eucalyptus** oil onto a Kleenex and to inhale. After her shower and few cups of basil tea, she was already feeling better. After inhaling the **eucalyptus** oil, she felt a great measure of relief in her blocked nose.

Now, in order to continue the effective treatment and try to prevent the other members of the household from catching the cold, it is a good idea to place 12 drops of one to three of the above oils in an oil burner. Besides the relief afforded by the inhalation of the essential oil vapors, they can also disinfect the house.

Denise attacked the cold from all sides by drinking tea, taking vitamin C, inhaling **eucalyptus** from a Kleenex, permeating the house with **eucalyptus**, **lemon**, and **basil** vapors by using an oil burner, resting, and even by using a special tip that a unique healer revealed to me – sucking on a purified garnet. After the stone has been purified (if it is new, two to three hours in salt water, and 24 hours outside or on the window sill. If it was not bought recently, it is enough to purify it on a crystal colony), it is placed in the mouth (preferably when the first signs of the cold appear), and sucked like a sweet for about two hours. Then it is rinsed well, placed on the purifying crystal colony for about two hours, and returned to the mouth and sucked once more. Amazing as this sounds, it works wonderfully, just like an antibiotic.

Because of the intensive treatment and Denise's wisdom, which told her that she had to stop running around – it was time to take a long rest – her cold passed easily within a few days.

Treating children and infant diseases with essential oils

Treating children's diseases with essential oils often has superb results. The reaction of the tots is very quick – frequently much quicker than that of adults. Having said that, it is very important to remember that there are many essential oils that are absolutely forbidden when it comes to treating infants and children, and others that are considered too powerful for them. Before we treat children and infants, it is mandatory to consult the chapter on warnings and ensure that we have not chosen one of the oils that is unsuitable for the treatment of children.

In aromatherapy for children, it is a good idea to stick to those oils that are known to be suitable for children and infants. They must be diluted in a very large amount of carrier oil compared to the usual dilution rate.

The oils that are recommended for the treatment of children and infants are: **chamomile, lavender, myrtle, niaouli, neroli, frankincense, mandarin** and **sandalwood**.

Under no circumstances must **sage, fennel, marjoram, myrrh, dill, lemongrass, cinnamon, red thyme,** *or* **eucalyptus** *be used in the treatment of children.* (**Sweet thyme** has a lower level of toxicity, and can be used with children over five.)

The dilution of the essential oils in carrier oils must be performed meticulously. When we treat an adult, the proportion is one drop of essential oil to 2 cc of carrier oil (that is, the essential oil is "half" of the amount of oil in the blend). When we treat big children, up to age 12, we use half the amount of essential oil. In other words, for 40 cc of carrier oil, we use 10 drops of essential oil. For little children, up to age six or seven, we prepare a blend in which we use a quarter of the amount of essential oils, that is, for 40 cc of carrier oil, we use five drops of essential oil. For infants of up to two years, we use less than an eighth of the amount of essential oil, that is, for 40 cc of carrier oil, we use two drops of essential oil. Moreover, we must pay attention that when a child is weak or small for his age, the amount of essential oil must be decreased.

Stomach pains caused by the accumulation of gas in children and infants

Linda, a teacher and the mother of 14-month-old twin girls, came to me with a very common complaint. Her two daughters, happy, healthy and lively babies, often suffered from stomach pains and flatulence as a result of gas accumulation. Her pediatrician explained that during the period when the babies were trying different kinds of solid food for the first time – such as cheese, mashed vegetables, puréed fruit and so on – this problem was very common and normal. At the same time, they were babies suffering from the problem, and Linda was looking for a natural, healthy, and suitable solution that would make it easier for them during the period of adapting to the new food.

The problem of gas accumulation among infants and tots is very widespread. It can be caused by the incorrect digestion and absorption of food, by the transition from mother's milk to milk substitutes, or by the transition from liquid food to solid food. Furthermore, it could be a symptom of an intolerance for or allergy to various foods (a very common complaint to which attention must be paid!) or a result of other individual factors.

I asked Linda to pay attention to the new foods the twins were receiving. I recommended that she not add more than one new food to their regular food every three to four days. When she added the new solid food – for instance, mashed chicken – she was to pay attention to any unusual phenomena in the twins' behavior for the next few days in order to see whether the problem of gas accumulation and stomach pains increased. She was to observe their behavior to see whether the new food was causing any changes. In this way, she could identify foods that could cause intolerance or allergies.

In addition, I prepared a special blend of essential oils for babies. In a 30-cc bottle, I used 28 cc of **almond** carrier oil, and 2 cc of **olive** oil. As we remember, when treating infants of up to two, we use about one-eighth of the regular amount of the essential oils. The regular amount of essential oil for 30 cc of carrier oil is 15 drops of essential oil. For this reason, in this case, we place only two drops of essential oil in the carrier oil. The essential oils I chose for treating the twins' problem were **lavender** and **chamomile**. I used one drop of each. As mentioned previously, **lavender** and **chamomile** are excellent oils for the general treatment of infants. They are excellent for the problem of stomach pains resulting from gas accumulation in general (for adults, too), and in the treatment of infants, they are the first choice of oils, since **lavender** is a very gentle oil that nevertheless has a multi-system effect (that is, it is suitable for treating various physical systems), and has a powerful effect on the immune system, which, in infants and young children, is not yet well-developed. **Chamomile** oil is superb for treating general problems of the digestive system and problems of gas accumulation, and it is also a very soothing and gentle oil.

We administer the essential oils via a very gentle massage, almost a spreading movement of the oils on the babies' abdomens, using light, circular movements, for less than 10 minutes. The massage must be performed every time the baby suffers from gas accumulation or stomach pains.

Linda tried the treatment the first time one of the twins had stomach pains. Her first impression was that the massage itself plus the fragrance of the oils caused the baby to calm down quickly and stop crying. Moreover, she mentioned that after the massage, the baby fell asleep easily, and had a very relaxed afternoon nap. A few hours later, when she woke up, she still had stomach pains – discomfort and restlessness – and Linda repeated the massage, but for a shorter time. She spread the oil over her abdomen with caressing movements for about five minutes, and watched her child calm down rapidly.

Lavender and **chamomile** oil, besides being very effective in the treatment of stomach pains, are both very soothing oils, and therefore, in the treatment of infants, we obtain two important results: soothing the baby, which results in the cessation of crying on the one hand, and relief of the stomach pains because of the action of the oils on the other.

Another treatment that is recommended for problems of stomach pains and gas accumulation in infants, is giving them chamomile tea to drink, preferably before the massage. In general, chamomile tea, which many infants who have not become accustomed to sweetened juice or tea can drink as it is, unsweetened, is an excellent tea for infants and children, and is a superb substitute for various sweetened juices or (regular) sweet tea for infants. It helps relieve stomach pains as a result of changes in diet or as a result of gas accumulation. It also soothes sensitive babies and facilitates sleep.

Lice

Every year, when the school year starts, I find myself swamped with calls from anxious mothers and fathers, parents of children in playschools, kindergartens, or the lower grades of elementary schools. Over and over again I hear the same question: What can be done in order to prevent the child from becoming infested with lice? What medication does the naturalist physician prescribe for this condition? Many parents are reluctant to shampoo their young children's heads with synthetic and chemical substances. Very fortunately, in recent years, a number of natural substances for treating lice have come onto the market. They are highly recommended because their level of toxicity is much lower than that of the chemical substances.

Lice are parasites that are nourished by sucking blood. In various countries, lice are an actual plague, but here, fortunately, it is head lice that are known, while body and pubic lice (known colloquially as "cooties") are less common. Contagion by head lice occurs mainly in kindergartens and schools. When children play together, their heads often come into contact, and the lice "jump" onto the clean head and begin to lay their eggs. Lice do not fly, so it requires actual head-to-head contact in order to be infected by them.

As many parents know, it is impossible to prevent the child from becoming infected while he is at school or kindergarten. Such admonitions as "Be careful not to get your head close to other children so you don't catch lice" are useless, since children tend to forget such warnings in the heat of play, and the unnecessary fear can cause them to keep away from certain children or to develop disproportionate fears about lice. Moreover, many mothers tend to become hysterical or overly panicked. These reactions only harm the child and scare him. Unfortunately, they do not scare or deter the lice…

The first step in treating lice is prevention – in other words, not to reach the frustrating stage of having to comb the child's head with a fine-toothed comb while he's screaming because you're pulling his hair, and you're revolted by the lice you've unearthed, not to mention the exhausting job of getting rid of all the eggs.

In order to prevent an infestation of lice, it is a good idea to place two to three drops of **rosemary** or **tea tree** oil into the shampoo used by the child. When this preventive action is taken for a long time, the essential oil that is dripped into the shampoo should be changed every few months. The oil must be mixed into the shampoo, shaking the bottle gently, and then the child's head must be shampooed according to the required frequency. Many families reported that since taking this preventive action, there are no more lice at home. From my professional experience, it was **rosemary** oil that won the majority of the praise, but **tea tree** oil was also found to be effective.

When an infestation does occur, there is no need to panic. The lice are not dangerous; they are simply a nuisance and must be gotten rid of quickly. The first stage is to check the child's head as soon as he complains of itching. In general, the moment the parents are informed of an infestation of lice at the kindergarten or school, the child's head must be checked every day when he gets home, since some children are less sensitive to itching and may complain only when their heads are already full of lice. It is important to look for the eggs, which are the source of the problem, in the region of the nape and ears, which are the favorite places for egg-laying. The eggs are very similar to dandruff, but, in contrast to dandruff, which can be shaken from the hair easily, louse eggs stick to it and are not so easy to remove. After the lice have been found, the lice and the eggs can be combed out using a special comb for this purpose. Then the head must be shampooed with special shampoo for treating lice. Before using the shampoo, however, it is worthwhile trying to treat the lice with essential oils. This treatment requires attention, since the action of the essential oils, as opposed to chemical substances, can differ from person to person. The treatment must be administered simultaneously to all the members of the household who are afflicted with lice in order to prevent a recurring infestation.

First of all, the head must be shampooed with shampoo that contains two or three drops of either **rosemary** or **peppermint** oil. After this, the hair must be towel-dried but still damp. To each person's head, apply a blend consisting of a tablespoon of **peanut** carrier oil, two drops of **rosemary** oil, and two drops of **geranium** oil. The blend must be spread over the entire head, and the head must be massaged slightly in order to get the oil to penetrate and to ensure that all the layers of hair are evenly covered. In cases of very long hair, it is possible to double the amount of oils in the blend. After spreading, cover the hair with a towel, and a polyethylene bag can be placed over the towel. Leave the blend on the hair for several hours – the longer the better –preferably all night. After removing the towel, the hair must be rinsed well – it can be washed once again with the shampoo containing the **rosemary** or **tea tree** oil – and begin combing the hair with the fine-toothed comb in order to remove the eggs and the dead lice. It is very important to launder the child's clothes and bed-linen very well and to thoroughly clean the brushes and combs that have come into contact with his hair over the last few days.

Impetigo

My neighbor, Rita, called me one Saturday afternoon, very upset, and asked me to come and see what had happened to her four-year-old son, Brett. Under Brett's chin and around his mouth there were clusters of little red blisters. Brett himself felt fine. His mood was not as good and amenable as usual, however, and the restlessness that stems from the disease could be discerned, but he continued playing without being overly concerned. Although he felt relatively good, the disease he had contracted had to be treated without delay.

Brett had contracted impetigo, which is a contagious skin disease that occurs in adults as well, but is more common in children. It is a bacterial skin infection that can appear anywhere on the skin, but is most common around the mouth. Sometimes the infection also reaches the neck and the scalp, and in certain cases even reaches other regions of the body. The disease manifests itself in slightly swollen rashes. Gradually, small blisters appear on a limited area of the skin, and burst after a while, revealing an area of red, moist, and oozing skin beneath them. After the liquid is expelled from the blisters, the infection spreads and is liable to move to other parts of the body, as well as infect other people. After the blisters burst, they become covered with yellowish scabs.

Although the disease can look very distasteful, it is not dangerous, unless it appears in newborns. In that case, it can jeopardize the infant's health.

Since impetigo is a contagious disease, the child must remain at home until the disease passes. He must use his own personal towel and bed-linen in order to prevent the infection spreading to the rest of the family. It is very important to seek medical attention, in parallel to aromatherapy, in order to prevent the spread of the disease in its full virulence. In general, the physician prescribes an antibiotic medication for treating the disease. When the disease is very severe, and the yellow scabs appear, it is important to wash them gently with water and disinfectant soap, dry the skin gently with a clean towel, which, of course, will be laundered immediately afterwards. The scabs must not be wiped vigorously or scratched.

The first step, of course, was to calm Rita down. She had panicked a bit at the thought of her son's contagious disease, which was unfamiliar to her. I explained the preventive measures she had to take, and I suggested that she go and see the doctor on Monday morning. In the meantime, it was important that

Brett receive the supportive aromatherapy treatment. The treatment would help stop the progress of the disease to the next stages. When treating more serious cases of impetigo, the treatment brings a great deal of relief. In any event, it is important to consult with a doctor and to take the medications, since, as I said before, the disease is liable to spread to other areas of the skin and infect other people as well.

The blend I prepared for Brett included 5 cc of **apricot kernel** oil, 5 cc of **wheatgerm** oil, and the following essential oils: two drops of **tea tree** oil, which is one of the most powerful antiseptic oils; two drops of **marigold** oil, which possesses properties that kill bacteria and fungi, soothe, and is especially suitable for very sensitive skin; and one drop of **geranium** oil, which is suitable for the treatment of a large variety of skin problems and infections and for Brett's irritated and sensitive skin. (Since the treatment is local, and Brett was a strong, healthy boy, I decided to use the adult dosage in this case.)

I asked Rita to apply the blend to the infected areas once or twice a day, and have Brett stay at home until the disease passed, so that he would not infect other children at kindergarten. Moreover, I suggested that she ask Brett's older siblings, who loved to spoil, hug, and kiss their little brother whenever they could, to understand that Brett was ill with an infectious disease at the moment, and they should not smother him with kisses, as they usually did.

The treatment with essential oils was extraordinarily helpful in preventing the spread of the disease and moderating its virulence. On Monday, when they went to see the pediatrician, there were still blisters, but just around his mouth and chin, and they were still at the initial stage, thanks to the aromatherapy, which prevented the spread and development of the blisters. Brett was given antibiotics, and Rita continued to apply the blend of essential oils to the infected areas of his skin once or twice a day for the following days. Three days later, the blisters disappeared without a trace. I recommended that Rita continue applying the oil to the area once a day for the next two days in order to ensure that nothing remained of the bacterial infection.

There are adults who are in the habit of using aromatherapy as a substitute for conventional medical treatment, but in this disease, it is important to be examined by a physician and to consult with him. When children are involved, twice as much care must be taken.

Aromatherapy for the skin

For thousands of years, essential oils – whether produced by contemporary methods or by more ancient ones – have had a far-reaching effect on skin care. For years, essential oils have been used in the cosmetics industry, starting from herbal baths containing essential oils, which were part of the daily skin care routine of noble and royal women in the ancient world, and up to the use of essential oils in today's cosmetics and perfumes.

The reward justifies the investment! Because of their wonderful fragrance, essential oils have always been the first choice for skin care and beauty treatment, and because of their marvelous properties and effects on body and mind alike, they have proved themselves to be effective in far-reaching ways in caring for the skin, for its nutrition, for maintaining its health, and for preventing its aging.

On the one hand, essential oils serve pure cosmetic purposes, and on the other, they have been found to be most effective for treating various skin problems, both chronic and acute.

From this chapter onward, we will relate to the oils as cosmetic skin nurturers, and we will also examine their beneficial effect on the treatment of various skin diseases.

When we treat the skin, and especially when we prepare an essence whose purpose is skin care, nutrition, and preservation, it is very important to relate to the type of skin. Both the carrier oils and the essential oils can be divided into oils that are suitable for the various skin types, according to three main groups: oils that are suitable for normal skin, oils that are suitable for dry skin, and oils that are suitable for oily skin. In addition, there are oils that are suitable for treating especially sensitive skin, for skin with a low level of moisture (not dry), for red skin, for wrinkled and aging skin, and so on.

Normal skin

This is the most common type of skin. It can be identified by its appearance – skin that is elastic, has a good level of vitality, is balanced in its secretion of sebum and perspiration, looks good, young, and not wrinkled, except for the usual expression lines.

In general, the T region – the bridge of the nose and the forehead – is shinier and greasier than the rest of the face.

Most of the carrier oils are suitable for normal skin, as are most of the essential oils.

Oily skin

Oily skin can be identified by the very shiny and greasy appearance of the surface of the skin. The shine and the oiliness stem from an imbalance between the sebaceous glands as well as from the fact that the sweat glands work more than usual. Oily skin can appear without pimples and blackheads in a condition in which there is over-secretion of the sebaceous glands, but the secretion is not thick. In contrast, there are many cases in which in addition to the oiliness of the skin, pimples, blackheads, and so on develop. This is characterized by an excessive and thick secretion, which, because of its thickness, gets stuck in the pores, accumulates, and becomes a pimple with an inflammation around it. When treating oily skin of this kind, we have to relate, in addition to the treatment with oils, to the person's nutrition. Of course, he has to be advised to immediately reduce the amount of saturated fat he consumes in fried foods or in animal fats, and to rectify the specific defects in his diet.

Generally, the suitable carrier oils for treating oily skin are **sesame** oil, **almond** oil (which dries the skin slightly), and **grapeseed** oil. It is possible to add **wheatgerm** oil or vitamin E to the blend.

The essential oils that are known to be especially suitable for treating oily skin are **myrrh**, **cypress** (which is mainly suitable for treating oily skin with pimples), **bergamot**, **lemon**, **chamomile**, and **tea tree**.

As we said before, when treating any kind of problem using aromatherapy, we do not make do only with the oils that are directly suitable for the problem, but also relate to the different factors and to the different problems involved in it, in order to attack the problem from all sides. When we treat oily skin using essential oils, we have to use oils whose properties also include the following: balancing sebum secretion, accelerating the expulsion of waste from the skin, and circulation and purification. When the skin is covered with pimples or infected pimples, we also look for anti-inflammatory oils and soothing oils. Moreover, we pay attention to the immune system, and try to ensure that the blend contains one of the oils that help reinforce it. When we look at the properties of the oils that are suitable for oily skin, we discover that many of them have additional properties that are necessary for treatment.

Cypress oil is also antiseptic, astringent, and shrinking; it heals pimples, knits tissues, and balances. **Bergamot** oil reinforces the immune system, is anti-inflammatory, soothes and balances the skin, and is good for treating open pores. **Chamomile** oil, which contains a relatively large quantity of starch, is a very effective anti-inflammatory oil; it is antiseptic, soothing, balancing, acts as a tonic for all the systems, and is especially suitable for allergic phenomena, and for all kinds of itches. It is very good for treating oily skin, itching, and allergies in infants. **Ylang ylang** oil, with its wonderful fragrance, is a marvelous oil for treating the skin. It balances the secretion of sebum, is good for oily skin with open pores, and soothes the skin. **Lemon** oil is a powerful antiseptic, good for treating open pores, and effective in causing spots and scars to fade. **Myrrh** oil is effective for oily skin with open pores; it is anti-inflammatory, a powerful antiseptic, and a good regenerator (renews cells and tissues). **Lavender** oil, too, can be included in the blend for treating oily skin. This oil is anti-inflammatory, a powerful antiseptic, an effective regenerator, and helps reinforce the immune system; it is also very effective on the emotional plane and has a large number of properties that are effective in almost all the body's systems, so that it often finds a place in various blends.

Sage oil, *which cannot be used by pregnant women*, (in fact, because of its high level of toxicity, it is recommended that only experienced professionals use it), can be effective in the blend as a stimulating, antiseptic astringent; it is a good regenerator and a tonic for all the body's systems. Moreover, it has an astringent affect, and is therefore good for treating acne. Having said that, because of the caution that its use requires, its relative, **clary sage**, which has a lower level of toxicity, may be safer and more correct for use (although *it must not be used during pregnancy*). **Clary sage** oil is a soothing oil that helps circulation and balances the secretion of sebum – for that reason, it is suitable for oily skin and also good for treating oily scalps.

Dry skin

The problem of dry skin is more common in women than in men because this condition can be influenced by the hormonal system. Dry skin frequently reflects a state of internal imbalance of the capillaries (the tiny blood vessels below the skin). The skin is constantly deficient; it does not receive an adequate and balanced blood supply, and the blood vessels do not expand, so less nutrition reaches the skin, and it becomes cold and dry. In such a condition, the skin looks dry and is prone to wrinkles. Sometimes deep wrinkles form. By touching the skin, it is possible to feel that the skin is rough and lacks elasticity, moisture, and vitality. In most cases, there are no blackheads on this type of skin and there is very low sebum secretion.

In treating dry skin, we use carrier oils that are considered "heavier," such as **olive** oil, which nourishes the skin very well because of the essential fatty acids it contains, **jojoba** oil, which prevents the escape of water from the skin, thus preserving its moistness, **avocado** oil, **wheatgerm** oil, **apricot** oil and **peach kernel** oil (because of their high quality).

The essential oils that are suitable for treating dry skin are **geranium, ylang ylang, jasmine, lavender, rosewater, neroli, cedarwood, frankincense, sandalwood, patchouli, clary sage, rose, orange** and **rosewood**.

Moreover, we will look for oils that fill the following requirements: give nutrients to the skin, stimulate circulation, regenerate and balance the sebum level (which, in contrast to oily skin, is too low). The carrier oils are generally responsible for the nutrition of the skin, because they contain a substantial quantity of minerals, vitamins, and essential fatty acids, as was described in the chapter on carrier oils.

To stimulate circulation, we can use **eucalyptus** oil, **lavender** oil, the luxurious **rose** oil with its marvelous fragrance, and **clary sage** oil. **Rose** oil is especially suitable when the skin is very sensitive or allergic.

Among the oils that balance the sebum level are **ylang ylang**, which balances the sebum level in dry skin very well, and **clary sage**. Among the powerful regenerators are the versatile **lavender** oil, **frankincense**, and **patchouli** with its special fragrance. (Some people are actually addicted to this fragrance, while others can't stand it. Therefore, it is a good idea to check with each client before including it in the blend.)

Neroli oil is a good regenerator for dry, old, wrinkled, and tired skin; it accelerates the growth of new cells and eliminates old cells.

Skin without moisture

Skin that lacks moisture looks like dry skin, but it is actually oily skin that has been "dried out" by incorrect nutrition, coffee, cigarettes, alcohol, severe weather conditions, and not drinking enough refreshing liquids. These things are likely to cause the production of thick, viscous sebum that gets stuck in the pores instead of passing through them. In cosmetic treatment of such a condition, we have to use moisturizing cosmetics, so we will work with oils that are suitable for normal and oily skin, and oils that are powerful regenerators. Of course, we will have to examine the nutritional aspects and deal with them accordingly. Carrier oils that are suitable for skin that lacks moisture are **sesame, grapeseed,** and **apricot**. It is advisable to add vitamin E and a small amount of **jojoba** oil to all the oils that are not very heavy.

The condition of skin that lacks moisture can also occur for a different reason. The use of soap and water or various cosmetic substances can dry out sensitive skin, and then an allergy occurs and the skin loses its moisture. In such a case, we choose essential oils that are suitable for sensitive skin such as **rose, chamomile,** and **lavender**. **Benzoin** oil, too, although it works slowly, has good qualities and is very effective in treating rashes and inflamed skin. **Melissa** oil, which is appropriate for the general treatment of allergies, can also be suitable for the problem.

Additional skin problems

There are other general conditions of the skin that require attention:

Skin with an uneven appearance – because of scars, blotches, freckles, and so on. **Lavender** oil is very suitable for creating an even look. **Lemon** and **rosewood** oils are known to make blotches and scars fade, and **fennel** oil is also suitable for treating blotches on the skin. In order to lighten the skin, use **lavender** and **lemon** oil as well as **sesame** carrier oil.

Congested skin – one of the following essential oils should be included in a blend: **basil, geranium, patchouli** or **rosemary**.

For treating *mature and old skin* – the essential oils **geranium, cypress, sandalwood, fennel, clary sage, vetiver,** and the carrier oil **jojoba** are suitable.

When the skin is also *wrinkled* – the following essential oils are highly recommended: **frankincense** (which is also effective in preventing the aging of the skin), **jasmine, neroli, chamomile** and **rose**.

Inflamed and red skin – the essential oils **angelica, benzoin, tea tree, jasmine, lavender, peppermint, cedarwood, petitgrain, patchouli,** and **rose**, and the carrier oil **grapeseed** are recommended. **Rosewater** is also suitable for use on sensitive, inflamed skin.

General strengthening of the skin – In order to maintain skin tone and elasticity, it is advisable to include one of the following oils in the blend, according to the needs of the person and his skin type: **juniper, geranium, myrrh, lemongrass, rose, basil, grapefruit, cypress, fennel, lemon,** or **frankincense**.

Refreshing the skin – For giving tired skin luster and vitality, it is advisable to include one or more of the following oils in cosmetic blends: **grapefruit, geranium, peppermint, neroli, rosemary, orange,** and **petitgrain**. **Avocado** carrier oil also contributes to refreshing the skin.

The preparation of cosmetics for skin care is not necessarily the ultimate solution for various skin problems. Skin problems, especially chronic ones, are usually directly linked to the person's general condition, and the emotional aspect has a primary significance in understanding the causes of skin problems. When treating skin problems, it is very important to pay attention to the person's emotional state. Moreover, we can give better treatment if we pay attention to the person's emotional state and express this concern in our choice of oils, when we prepare a "totally" cosmetic blend for care, nutrition, and improving the look of healthy skin: in addition to beautiful, healthy facial skin, the person also gains emotional well-being.

The appearance of the skin is an expression of a person's lifestyle. When he is under pressure, or leads an unhealthy life, eats junk food, is exposed to pollution, or has a problem in any of his systems, the signs of the irregularities and imbalances can be seen in various skin diseases and phenomena. Diseases such as jaundice manifest themselves in the skin. In jaundice, the skin takes on a yellow cast. In anemia, the skin is paler than usual. A lack of proper care for the body, or not drinking enough, can be expressed in tired, wrinkled, or dry skin. The state of the hormonal system may also be reflected in the skin, and we can discern a broad spectrum of states of hormonal imbalance from a few pimples preceding the menstrual period, via infected acne, to excessive hairiness. Frequently, skin problems indicate a problem in the immune system or an allergy, and the skin can help us to discern a general sensitivity of the body. (When the person is very allergic in his facial skin, it is advisable to check whether he has other allergies, and to examine his immune system.) Problems of lymphatic drainage and circulation can be expressed in congested skin and edemas. Allergies can be expressed in itching and rashes, as well as in fungal infections and eczema, which show us that something in the immune system is not operating smoothly. (The condition can stem from a mild imbalance to chronic ongoing weakness of the immune system. The frequency, duration, and intensity of the eczema or fungal infections provide us with information about this.)

Of course, when we try to understand the condition of the body according to the skin, we must not jump to premature conclusions. It is important to understand why the skin looks like it does, and, to that end, we must pose a set of questions (either to ourselves or to the client). It is important to know whether the client's lifestyle includes habits that harm his skin, such as smoking, imbibing alcohol, poor nutrition, and so on. These habits can weaken the immune system. Good sleep is also essential for the health of the skin. The consumption of a lot of fats, excessive cholesterol, and so on, will also manifest itself in the skin – for instance, oily skin with pimples. Intestinal problems, too, such as constipation, as well as a lack of proper cleansing and drainage in the body, are likely to manifest themselves in pimples and various skin rashes.

Likewise, it is important to find out if the person is undergoing any kind of supplementary treatment that is causing reactions of cleansing, such as reflexology, Bach flower remedies, and so on. In principle, every occurrence of pimples or a similar phenomenon that is not serious as a result of some kind of treatment (even hypnotism or psychotherapy) or cleansing or detoxifying work, which lasts for a few days, may result from toxins exiting the body via the skin, cleansing and invigorating the circulation, and other factors related to the treatment. In such a case, it is important to consult with the therapist and find out whether this is a reaction. In any event, skin phenomena can be relieved with aromatherapy. (If contact is made with another therapist, it is possible and advisable to work collaboratively with him/her.)

Another point that must be taken into account when preparing oils for treating skin problems or for skin care is as follows: it is not advisable to use several different oil blends in a treatment. As we said before, in general, a blend is made up of a maximum of four different oils. For a cosmetic treatment, it is a good idea to use the same oils that were used in the massage, oil burner, and bath. It is possible to mix those oils into a face tonic, face cream, and so on, but there should always be one basic blend. Luckily for us, every oil has so many different properties that with a little bit of work, we can find the perfect and unique treatment for each person. It is true that the use of general "recipes" for treatment will also lead to good results, so long as we take the counter-indications and warnings into account (see chapter on warnings), but the more we match the treatment to each individual client, the more in-depth the treatment will be. Make no mistake – a comprehensive and in-depth aromatherapy treatment can have an effect that is stunning in its intensity, from the physical, emotional, and esthetic points of view. Of course, the oils also have an energetic and spiritual effect, but that is another topic altogether.

Mature skin

Moira, the 52-year-old director of a marketing company and mother of three grown children, came for cosmetic treatment with aromatherapy in order to improve her facial skin. Moira had been using various face creams for a long time, but 30 years of smoking and continuous and disproportionate exposure to the summer sun had made her skin look lifeless, old, and rather baggy. The creams she used sometimes improved the look of her skin, but did not achieve the desired results.

Cosmetic treatment of mature skin is administered by beauticians only, but anyone can prepare a blend of nourishing and cleansing oils and use it for massaging the facial skin, reviving it, and giving it luster, freshness, and a general "youthful" appearance.

In general, the essential oils that are suitable for mature or old skin are **geranium, cypress, sandalwood, fennel, clary sage, vetiver, frankincense** (which is also effective in preventing skin aging), **jasmine, neroli, chamomile**, and **rose**. The last five oils are also very effective for wrinkled skin.

The carrier oils that are suitable for treating this kind of skin are **jojoba, cherry kernel**, and **borage**. **Apricot kernel** oil, which is a superb cosmetic oil, is also suitable for treating mature skin, preferably with the addition of one of the other carrier oils.

For Moira's treatment, I chose to use **jojoba, apricot kernel**, and **borage** carrier oils. From the essential oils, I chose **frankincense, patchouli**, and a little **rosemary** oil.

The first stage of treatment was to cleanse Moira's face of all traces of makeup and dirt. I used pure **almond** oil for this purpose. (This cleansing can be done at home, since it is simple. It is also possible to use **almond** oil as a natural substitute for face lotion for cleansing the skin and residual makeup.) First, I spread the almond oil over Moira's face, using gentle cleansing movements: using my fingers, from the center of the forehead outward toward the eyebrows and around the eyes, going down to the bridge of the nose, spreading the oil on it and on the sides of the nose, outward, and to the cheeks, using both palms. Remember that the movements go toward the sides of the face. The chin is massaged with oil in the same way as the forehead – starting in the middle, and spreading the oil outward along the chin and lower jaw with the fingers, below the chin and onto the neck. After spreading the oil, I took a piece of cotton and removed the oil in exactly the same manner I had applied it, taking care to clean off every area. The excellent results of the cleansing could be seen in the brown dirt on the cotton.

Afterwards, I prepared a facial mask from a gel (which can be prepared from a powder that is obtainable in the appropriate stores). Two drops of **eucalyptus** oil are added to the gel in order to improve its action. After spreading the gel on Moira's face, I placed gauze on the layer of gel and on them I placed a compress made of a felt mask soaked in **rosewater**. (To prepare the compress, use two drops of **rosewater** in two cups of water.) I covered the felt mask with plastic wrap (leaving openings for the nose and mouth, of course) and left it on for about 15 minutes.

After that time, I removed the mask and cleansed Moira's face well. Then I began the massage with nourishing oil that I prepared from 5 cc of **jojoba** carrier oil, 5 cc of **apricot kernel** carrier oil, and five drops of **borage** oil. I added the following essential oils to the blend of nourishing carrier oils: two drops of **frankincense**, two drops of **patchouli**, and one drop of **rosemary**. Via massage, the oils penetrated Moira's skin well. It is important to remember that in cases of treating mature skin with broken capillaries, **achillea** or **parsley** oil must be used instead of **patchouli**.

After the cosmetic treatment, Moira was surprised at the initial improvement in her facial skin. Her skin looked cleaner, smoother, and softer, and its general appearance was healthier and more glowing. I recommended that she use **almond** oil for cleansing her skin every day, and massage her face with nourishing oil every night before going to sleep. Moira performed the cleansing and the massage meticulously and reported that the state of her skin had improved enormously. It was smoother and more pliant, elastic, and glowing.

Cracked skin

Shelly, a 35-year-old mother of three, wanted an effective alternative to using hand cream, which she did not like, in order to treat the cracked skin of her hands. According to her, although the hand cream she used was of good quality, it helped the condition for a few hours only, and she wanted a treatment that would nourish the skin of her hands more significantly.

Cracked skin occurs mainly in the winter and in people who work regularly with various chemical substances such as cleaning materials. Cracked skin occurs mainly in the hands, and sometimes in the feet. Occasionally, this condition may stem from various skin ailments, and then, of course, in addition to aromatherapy for the cracked skin, it is advisable to treat the disease itself. In certain cases, as in Shelly's, the problem of cracked skin can be very disturbing, and can cause discomfort, when every movement of the fingers causes an annoying pain. Generally, it is advisable and very important for people who come into contact with various chemical substances such as bleach, dishwashing liquid and the like to avoid the harmful effect of the substances on their skin by using rubber gloves into which talcum powder has been sprinkled.

When cracked skin is caused by the cold, it is important to put on warm gloves before going outside into the cold winter weather. Likewise, it is important to massage the skin with products that provide the skin with moisture, and not to wash the hands too often, since frequent washing aggravates the situation and the pain.

The treatment I prepared for Shelly is very effective for cracked skin, and can be used many times throughout the day in order to soothe the pain and restore moisture and pliancy to the skin. The blend for treating cracked skin can be prepared from 25 cc of **peanut** oil, 5 cc of **wheatgerm** oil, and 15 drops of **geranium** essential oil. I recommended that Shelly apply the blend every time she felt the need, and should try to leave the blend on her hands as long as possible.

Shelly tried the blend and greatly enjoyed the feeling of moisture and pliancy it provided. In the beginning, she applied the blend to her hands frequently during the day, but gradually, after a week of constant use, she began to see a significant improvement in the state of the skin of her hands. The skin became more pliant. Previously red and cracked, it now looked better and regained its elasticity. She needed treatment less frequently, but she still took care to apply the blend to her hands at least once a day in order to nourish the skin and maintain the results she had achieved.

Stretch marks

Sandie, a good-looking, well-groomed woman of 28, came for aromatherapy treatment for a reason that was basically cosmetic. She worked as head accountant in a large organization, and generally attributed a great deal of importance to her external appearance. She had been married for five years, and was the mother of a three-and-a-half-year-old daughter and a four-month-old son. Already after her first pregnancy, Sandie had noticed stretch marks, which bothered her, especially during the summer, when she wanted to wear a swimsuit that showed off her shapely body at the beach and the pool. She told me that she had lost the weight she had gained during the pregnancies very easily, since she had a slim build by nature, and had taken up vigorous sporting activity in order to get her body back into shape and get rid of the stretch marks. Moreover, she used various cosmetics that claimed to help get rid of stretch marks, but they only helped minimally.

After her second pregnancy, deep, red stretch marks appeared over her bottom, abdomen, thighs, and chest. The marks gradually became grayish-yellow. At this point, her special exercises and cosmetic creams were hardly of use to her, and she suffered from a great deal of mental anguish.

During our interview, I asked Sandie to describe her daily diet, which turned out to be healthy and normal, and provided her body and skin with the basic food, minerals, and vitamins required for post-pregnancy regeneration. She mentioned that during and after the pregnancy, she had consulted with a dietician and an orthomolecular specialist, and had received guidelines for the food supplements necessary for her body. When I asked her if she suffered from any other symptoms, physical or emotional, she explained that her general physical condition was satisfactory, except for the fact that she tended to get ill three or four times during the winter with viral infections. She did not think too much about this, however, since, as she said, "everyone gets ill and becomes infected during the winter." When I went into this more deeply, she admitted that she was under great pressure at work, found it hard to relax, even after work, because of her horribly heavy schedule – which included an eight-hour work day, devoting time to her daughter and infant son and taking care of them, and participating in several activities, classes and courses – and was in a state of stress most of the time, and only late at night, toward bedtime, did she allow herself to relax a little, watch TV, read the newspaper or rest.

Although Sandie's main complaint was the stretch marks, in aromatherapy it is necessary to relate to all of the client's symptoms and in this case, Sandie's immune system was not in optimal condition. (Luckily for Sandie, she took essential food supplements, exercised regularly, and had an optimistic nature and a lot of vitality, and this greatly decreased the damage to her immune system.) It was almost certain that her condition stemmed from the constant stress she was under. For this reason, the oils I chose for treating Sandie were oils with a triple effect: skin treatment – that is, regenerative oils (that stimulate renewed growth); astringent oils for shrinking the stretch marks, and, at the same time, with a calming effect, for treating the stress she was under on a daily basis; moreover, it was important to include at least one oil with a beneficial, reinforcing effect on the immune system.

The oils I chose for treating Sandie were **apricot kernel**, **wheatgerm**, and **borage** carrier oils, and **lavender**, **frankincense**, and **neroli** essential oils. It must be mentioned that Sandie had a tendency toward sensitive skin.

Since the problem under discussion is mainly a cosmetic one (despite the hormonal connection), the carrier oils I selected were blatantly cosmetic oils. **Apricot kernel** oil, the main carrier oil in the blend, was chosen because in addition to its property of being absorbed quickly in the skin, it also improves the skin's elasticity and maintains its moisture. Besides these properties, it is considered to be mainly a cosmetic oil, since it helps with the regeneration of the skin cells, it is rich in vitamin A, and it is of extremely high quality. (For this reason, it is expensive, and you must pay attention, when purchasing it, that it really is authentic and quality **apricot kernel** oil, and not be tempted to buy ineffective and sometimes harmful substitutes!) The **borage** oil has regenerative properties (that is, it helps renew the skin cells) as well as a high GLA content, which also helps with conditions linked to the hormonal system. In the case of stretch marks, this oil can be exchanged for **rose-hip** or **calendula** oil (it is important to ensure that the latter is 100% cold-pressed!), which help greatly in treating stretch marks. The additional oil in the blend of carrier oils was **wheatgerm** oil, which is rich in vitamin E and is used as a natural anti-oxidant, and as such helps maintain the quality of the blend and preserves it for a long time. If we are already talking about **wheatgerm** oil, it is important to mention that it cannot be used as the main carrier oil in a blend, because it is very heavy and has a dominant odor. However, it is a good idea to add a few drops of it to the blend in order to utilize its anti-oxidant effect, which, besides its effectiveness in application and its importance for the skin, also preserves the blend by protecting it from oxidation.

I chose **lavender** oil because of its very powerful properties. In fact, there is hardly any problem this oil cannot treat. Add to this its especially low level of toxicity, the ease of obtaining it, and its relatively low price, together with the fact that it can be used for treating children and the elderly (something that cannot be done with oils that have a high level of toxicity), and you have an oil that is a must in every first-aid closet! **Lavender** oil is wonderful for treating a variety of skin problems. In our blend, for treating Sandie's stretch marks, it provided its well-known effect of soothing the skin and helped regenerate the skin cells. In addition, **lavender** oil is excellent for general calming of body and mind and for use in situations of stress, and reinforces the immune system, so it met our needs – in Sandie's case – to help dispel and calm the stress she was under, and help reinforce her immune system.

Frankincense oil is wonderful for treating stretch marks because of its good regenerative properties and its help in smoothing wrinkles. In addition, it is a soothing, effective, and pleasant oil.

Neroli oil, like **frankincense** and **lavender** oil, is a very soothing oil, and excellent for treating stretch marks.

To prepare the blend, I used 20 cc of **apricot kernel** oil, 5 cc of **wheatgerm** oil, and 5 cc of **borage** oil. I added five drops of **lavender** oil, five drops of **frankincense**, and five drops of **neroli** to the blend of carrier oils.

I asked Sandie to perform a gentle massage on the areas where the stretch marks occurred – on her abdomen, breasts, and thighs – once a day.

Sandie told me that the treatment and massage with essential oils was very enjoyable and gave her a good feeling. However, only after two weeks of treatment did she begin to see results – the stretch marks began to be less noticeable and it seemed that in certain areas they had faded substantially. I recommended that she continue with the daily treatment until she obtained the desired results.

Getting stretch marks to fade can take some time, sometimes even several months – this depends on the client, her skin, her nutrition, and the extent of her physical activity. In Sandie's case, after three months of treatment, her stretch marks faded almost totally, and the following summer, after the aromatherapy and her stringent exercise regimen, she could already go to the beach in a skimpy swimsuit.

Spider veins (broken capillaries)

Julia, a 28-year-old cosmetics salesperson, came to my clinic looking well-groomed and smelling of expensive perfume. She was hoping that aromatherapy would provide her with a solution to her problem of spider veins. She had tried various creams, but the problem had not disappeared. Her general state of health was very good, and she did not suffer from any other problems, but she mentioned that she had a very sensitive nature, and sometimes, before her period, she was hypersensitive, tense, and almost depressed.

Julia's facial skin had always been very sensitive, fair, and delicate. Broken capillaries in the face are a problem that is well known to many people with sensitive skin. Very thin veins appear on the surface of the cheeks and nose, spreading over the area in a manner that is reminiscent of a spider web. Generally speaking, spider veins is a network of weak veins through which the blood can be seen, and they are liable to appear in other areas in the body where the skin is delicate and sensitive, such as the neck and the back of the hands. Sometimes, they characterize reddish and congested skin.

When the skin is sensitive and there are broken capillaries in it, it is highly recommended that the person avoid exposure to the sun, use a suitable sunscreen, and avoid saunas and hot springs. Very hot baths, washing the face in hot water, or facial treatment with steam are not suitable for people with broken capillaries. Moreover, it is important to use cosmetics for sensitive skin, and cosmetics that are alcohol-free.

For general treatment, we use the following essential oils: **chamomile**, **rose**, **peppermint**, **cypress**, **parsley** and **achillea**.

As carrier oils, the following gentle cosmetic oils are suitable for treatment: **apricot kernel**, **cherry kernel**, and **peach kernel**.

For Julia, I prepared a mixture that included 10 cc of **apricot kernel** oil, one drop of **rose** oil, and two drops of **chamomile** oil, two essential oils that are very effective in the treatment of spider veins, as well is helping Julia's hypersensitivity, the tension and bad mood she suffered from because of the premenstrual hormonal changes in her body; I also added two drops of **parsley** oil, which is wonderful for treating spider veins.

The treatment was administered via a very gentle face massage with the blend, and took about 20 minutes. After the massage, I asked Julia to remain lying down for about 15 minutes in order to enable the oils to work optimally while she rested.

She felt marvelous after the first treatment. A facial massage, when it is done with intention, with gentle, full movements, using suitable oils that have a soothing effect and a pleasant smell, can be a truly sublime experience.

In addition to the pleasant experience, after three months of treatment once a week (with her applying the blend to her face every evening), Julia saw an enormous improvement in the condition of her capillaries. Most of them had disappeared, and her skin looked much more even. Its tone was also much better, and it felt and looked stronger and fresher.

After about five months of treatment, there were only a few capillaries left around Julia's nostrils, but almost all the capillaries that had discolored her cheeks had disappeared or faded.

Varicose veins

Sheena, a single, 32-year-old psychological counselor in an elementary school, came for aromatherapy because of a disturbing problem. Her health was good, but she was 33 pounds overweight. Despite her obesity, she took trouble with her grooming, made sure to be fashionable and elegant, and was even blessed with impressive beauty, which was emphasized by her daily grooming. However, she was bothered by one problem: for three years, she had suffered from varicose veins on her calves. The veins were swollen, protruding, and reddish-blue, and she was ashamed to wear a skirt or any other clothing that exposed her calves. The problem was not just esthetic. As a result of the varicose veins, Sheena suffered from pains in her legs and from swollen feet, and after a day of work, and for several days before her period, the swelling increased, as did the pains.

Varicose veins are a very common phenomenon, but much more so in women than in men. The disease is more common in people who stand for long periods of time, in pregnant women, in obese or tall people, or in people who have family histories of varicose veins. Varicose veins are actually swollen veins, usually in the leg, mainly in the inner part of the leg, but can be found anywhere on the leg, from the groin to the ankle. They occur as a result of a problem in the action of the valves of the veins. Normally, the blood in the legs returns to the heart, some of it via the action of the leg muscles. The shallow veins of the leg are involved in this process, as are the deep veins. The blood flows from the tissues of the leg to the shallow veins, which are near to the muscles, and via linking veins, it passes to the deep veins that are situated in the muscles. As a result of the person's movements, the leg muscles alternately relax and contract, and the deep veins and the linking veins spread and receive blood from the shallow veins. Inside the deep and linking veins there are valves that prevent the "used" blood from flowing back into the shallow veins. When the action of the valves of the deep veins is defective, the blood may be pushed back into the shallow veins, and as a result of the pressure to which they are subjected, the shallow veins twist and swell, and varicose veins are formed. Varicose veins protrude, are bluish and swollen, and the more the damaged vein protrudes on the surface of the skin, the more sensitive it becomes, and an itching sensation begins in the skin covering it. In such a condition, pains can spread all over the legs, the feet swell after prolonged standing, and sometimes the pains increase before and after menstruation.

In general, varicose veins are not dangerous, but are a painful nuisance. However, in rare cases, various complications can arise as a result of problems in the blood supply to the tissues, to the point of varicose ulcers. In cases of a varicose ulcer, *medical care must be sought immediately*. As treatment, elastic stockings are recommended. Sometimes, the physician suggests bandages that are soaked in analgesic substances in order to lessen the itching, similar to what is done in aromatherapy. In any event, it is important to stand as little as possible, and to sit with the legs on a footstool. In serious cases, the only solution to the problem is surgery, in which the damaged veins are extracted from the legs, but in 10 percent of cases, the varicose veins return and appear in another area on the leg.

When Sheena asked me to "solve" her varicose vein problem, I answered that with aromatherapy the chances of making her varicose veins disappear were very small. What was possible to do, very effectively, was to ease the pain, the irksome itching in the area, and possibly reduce the swelling. Sheena sometimes consulted with a dietician concerning a weight-loss program, and together, in a collaborative effort, losing weight and undergoing treatment with aromatherapy, her condition could be alleviated substantially.

The treatment with essential oils that was devised for Sheena was a massage treatment. As a carrier oil, I chose 10 cc of **apricot kernel** oil, to which I added two drops of **parsley** oil, one drop of **juniper** oil, one drop of **cypress** oil, and one drop of **peppermint** oil. I recommended that Sheena massage her legs once a day, performing upward massage strokes – in other words, in the direction of her heart.

After a week of massage, Sheena felt some relief from the pain and itching. She continued the treatment, and gradually the pain became less and less, the itching disappeared almost totally after applying the oils, and, at a certain stage, the swelling that would appear in her legs after a day's work went down and diminished. After three months of treatment, Sheena decreased the number of massages to three a week, and, after six months, she only needed two a week in order to relieve her condition. After a year of aromatherapy, and losing 18 pounds, the state of her varicose veins improved significantly, and the veins, which no longer caused her pain, barely protruded. Now she can camouflage them with pantihose or special makeup for hiding (regular) veins in the leg, and they are barely visible.

Cellulite

Karin, a 42-year-old computer expert and mother of four, worked hard to maintain her lovely figure. She was tall, with a broad build and a tendency to put on weight, and until about four years previously had suffered from obesity. After her last birth, five years before, she went on a balanced and healthy diet under a nutritionist's supervision, and from then on had lost weight. She worked out once a week in the gym, swam both in the pool and in the sea in the summer, and went power-walking twice a week for about an hour. Karin maintained a healthy, balanced diet that was low in calories and in animal protein, and took the appropriate food supplements. Despite her impressive weight loss and body strengthening via physical activity (she told me that since she started exercising, many problems in her life had been solved and her general health had improved beyond recognition), Karin suffered from cellulite that accumulated during the years she was overweight (since her youth), and they spoiled the nice figure she had acquired over the last years, thanks to correct nutrition and healthy physical activity.

Cellulite consists of areas in which the fat cells in the subcutaneous layer grow and swell and create hollows and protrusions, sometimes slightly rough, on the surface of the skin, mainly in the area of the buttocks and thighs. While cellulite often goes hand in glove with obesity, it can also appear in people who have a genetic tendency toward it or toward obesity (even if their weight is balanced), as well as in people who were once obese but lost weight. This is because the fatty tissue that causes cellulite begins to form at a young age, and "swells" over the years. For this reason, even after weight loss and physical exercise, deposits of cellulite can form over the surface of the thighs and buttocks. It is important to remember that the main cause of cellulite development is overeating and obesity, and for this reason it is important that the treatment relate to nutritional factors and general diet. Treating cellulite with aromatherapy is effective when it is combined with regular physical activity and with correct and healthy eating habits, and in the case of being overweight or obese, a suitable diet. In any event, the cellulite deposits can sometimes prove to be stubborn, and require ongoing and relentless physical exercise, diet, and aromatherapy treatments to get rid of them. The effectiveness and success of the treatment depend to a large extent on the client himself.

In Karin's case, she revealed a great deal of awareness of the problem, and her attitude toward nutritional balance and physical activity was good.

The essential oils that are suitable for treating cellulite are **grapefruit** (which is recommended generally for weight problems), **patchouli** and **fennel**, which are oils for treating obesity (**fennel** is known as an appetite repressant, and **patchouli** can repress appetite to a certain extent), **juniper, angelica, rosemary, thyme**, and **cinnamon** (which are stimulating and invigorating), **cypress** (which is an excellent astringent), **carrotseed**, and **lemon**. From this selection, I choose the oils that are suitable for the particular client's overall physical and emotional states. I also prefer to choose oils that are suitable for the client's skin. In the choice of carrier oils, too, I choose an oil according to how it suits the client's skin or the nature of his overall problems. When the treatment concentrates mainly on the problem of cellulite, I prefer **almond** oil.

The oils I chose for Karin's treatment were **rosemary, grapefruit, juniper**, and **cypress**. To a 30-cc bottle filled with **almond** carrier oil, I added three drops of **rosemary** oil, four drops of **grapefruit** oil, three drops of **cypress** oil, and four drops of **juniper** oil. I prepared the same blend of essential oils for her to use in the bath.

I recommended that Karin take an aromatic bath two to three times a week, dripping 4-5 drops of the blend of pure essential oils into it, and staying in the bath for about 20 minutes. It was a good idea for her to put on some soothing, calm, pleasant background music while she soaked in the warm, fragrant bath, and do abdominal breathing exercises. While it is true that the breathing exercises, the relaxation, and the pleasant music would not shrink the cellulite deposits, the total relaxation in the aromatic bath would give her vitality and a good feeling, and free her from tension and from everyday pressures. After the bath, she was to dry off gently, without rinsing or soaping herself, in order not to adversely affect the continuing action of the oils. After her body was dry, she was to apply some of the blend containing carrier oil onto the areas with the cellulite, massage them well, and rub and brush them with a suitable body brush. (Massage brushes with hard rubber bristles are available, and they are excellent for rubbing. In principle, however, any brush that facilitates the penetration of the oils into the body, performs the massage and rubbing action, and is also pleasant for the user, is suitable for the purpose.) I recommended that Karin perform the massage and the brushing every day after her shower (including the days she did not have an aromatic bath).

Karin persisted with the treatment for a long time. During the first months, she did not see much change in the cellulite deposits, although she certainly enjoyed the baths emotionally and physically, and felt that they were good for her skin. The massage and rubbing gave her a good feeling of blood flow and movement in the areas in which the cellulite deposits were located. Apparently, an improvement had begun, but it was still not visible. Six months after starting the treatment, Karin began to see clear results; she felt that the cellulite centers were shrinking, and that the protrusions had flattened somewhat. After a year of treatment, Karen was already wearing her swimsuit in which the protrusions of cellulite, that were once obvious and conspicuous, were flat and much smaller, and this contributed greatly to her lovely figure.

Skin diseases

There is a vast range of problems related to skin diseases. Among them, are chronic and acute problems, some of which are severe and troublesome and can be an esthetic or even functional liability (such as psoriasis), others that are more or less a "nuisance," while still others that tend to be ignored, and lived with (such as athlete's foot). The problems can be caused internally as a result of a lack of inner equilibrium – such as psoriasis, acne, and so on; or as the result of an internal reaction to an external factor – an allergic reaction – such as dermatitis, rashes, and infections, and even from external factors, such as burns, sunburn, injuries and blows (which we will deal with in the chapter on first aid).

Psoriasis vulgaris

Kim, 34 years old, came for aromatherapy treatment for the psoriasis that had broken out five years previously. Psoriasis is a chronic skin disease that appears in 2% of the population. The causes are not known. The disease is characterized by an uncontrolled cornification of the cells, generally in folds of skin – elbows, knees, buttocks. Under the outer layers of skin, layers of dried keratin are formed and there is no aeration – and this is what causes redness and infection. A scaliness accumulates in the following typical places: on the elbows, on the knees, and sometimes on the abdominal skin. There is also erythroderma – red skin with little bubbles. Sometimes, during an attack and when the condition is severe, infections can appear in these places because the skin is cracked. There is also a type of psoriasis that only appears on the soles of the feet and the palms of the hands.

Psoriasis is a disease of outbreaks and remissions. During an outbreak, there is a typical appearance – silver scales in the indicated places surrounded by red skin and vesicles. The disease may stem from several causes, so the treatment must be specific to the particular person, in order to identify the root of the problem – physical, spiritual, emotional, or mental.

The causes of the first appearance and of an outbreak of psoriasis: The disease can appear at any age, even in children. It has a hereditary component. It occurs when there is emotional stress, and more in the winter. The best treatment is UVA radiation, so it is recommended that someone with psoriasis spends as much time as possible at the Dead Sea in Israel, several times a year. The sojourn at the Dead Sea (which is famous for its successful treatment of psoriasis) provides relief for up to half a year. In severe cases, the disease is treated with steroids.

Treating psoriasis with aromatherapy entails a careful examination and the treatment of the emotional causes of the onset of the disease, since tension and emotional pressure exacerbate the symptoms. Today, there is as yet no method, natural or chemical, for curing the disease altogether. Using aromatherapy, it is possible to relieve and moderate the symptoms, and sometimes lead to longer intervals between outbreaks of the disease.

Kim worked as a telemarketing manager in a large company. While she was satisfied with her job, she was exposed to constant time pressure and worked long hours. In general, her overall state of health was good, she kept fit and stuck to a healthy diet. Two years previously, she began a macrobiotic diet, and she said that since then, the frequency of the outbreaks had decreased a bit. Kim suffered from psoriasis most months of the year, but in fall and winter, there was a massive increase in outbreaks. An outbreak of psoriasis means severe over-cornification of the skin in the places that are sensitive to the disease, and during winter and fall, the situation reached a point that Kim could hardly bend her elbows because of the over-cornification of the skin on them. A hard gray and reddish scaliness appeared on her knees and abdomen as well, causing her a great deal of suffering. The disease did not disappear altogether during the summer or when she spent a few weeks at the Dead Sea, but it did calm down. Having said that, Kim was interested in getting aromatherapy in order to alleviate her condition, especially in the fall and winter, since then it was really unbearable.

Psoriasis caused Kim a lot of suffering. She felt uncomfortable exposing her elbows, which were covered with reddish-gray horny and scaly skin, so she wore blouses that covered her elbows, even in the hot summer months. Of course, she did not wear miniskirts or shorts, either, because of her knees, which were covered with dry, scaly skin. Besides the physical discomfort, psoriasis is not esthetic and limits the sufferers in many ways. As I said before (and most unfortunately), there is as yet no treatment that can eliminate the disease altogether.

During my conversation with Kim, it transpired that the psoriasis had broken out initially during her divorce proceedings. It was winter, and her divorce, after seven years of marriage – with the struggle over property, child custody, and so on – caused her tremendous emotional stress and tension. All this went on while she continued going to work and taking care of her children as usual.

The outbreak of psoriasis after divorce is a common occurrence, and is almost certainly brought on by the constant tension. (However, tension does not cause the disease, which is apparently already present in the body in a dormant state, and breaks out in situations of stress and crisis.) The outbreak of the disease after divorce is so widespread that it has been nicknamed "the divorce disease."

Kim complained that now, after she had gotten divorced and was ready to begin a new life, this tiresome disease had struck. She admitted that she was ashamed to wear beachwear, and felt that the disease interfered with her meeting new men. Kim invested a great deal of energy in her work and in taking care of her children, and it was a shame that she was so disturbed by her external appearance and by the fact that other people would notice her disease. She also invested an enormous amount of energy and thought into ways of hiding the flaws on her skin. A shame, since everyone has different flaws, and if she were to accept herself as she was, it is almost certain that others would accept her, too.

Unfortunately, there is no "magic formula" for making psoriasis go away. Many studies have been published, but a medication that will cure the disease completely has not yet been found. The sufferers have to learn to live with their skin affliction, and try to ease and moderate the symptoms of the disease in different ways. Besides a sojourn at the Dead Sea – which is highly recommended for people who suffer from skin diseases – it is important for psoriasis patients to receive nutritional balance from an experienced professional, and orthomolecular treatment (treatment with food supplements, such as vitamins and minerals) that can achieve good results in treating the disease. Aromatherapy is very effective in easing and moderating the symptoms of the disease, but it produces different results in different individuals. In any event, it is worth trying, since it does not involve any great effort or expense, and can produce good results – sometimes even better than expected.

In aromatherapy, we treat psoriasis with general and local massage, baths, and the oil burner. The oils that are generally suitable for treating psoriasis are: **cedarwood, yarrow, ylang ylang, bergamot, sandalwood, juniper, tea tree, chamomile, lavender, geranium, peppermint,** and **achillea. Lavender, geranium,** and **chamomile** oils mainly relate to the treatment of the emotional aspect of the disease.

In the treatment of psoriasis, the carrier oils are of great importance. The carrier oils that are effective in treating psoriasis are: **wheatgerm, avocado, borage,** and **sesame.**

It is also possible to treat psoriasis with carrier oils only. This is done by preparing a blend from 10 ml **wheatgerm** oil, 10 ml **avocado** oil, 10 ml **sesame** oil, and 5 ml **borage** oil. This blend can be applied every morning and evening to the areas that are afflicted by the disease.

Better results may occur when the emotional side of the client is also treated, since in many people, this disease tends to become more severe or moderate in accordance with their emotional state. In any event, when it is a matter of an inflamed condition, such as Kim's condition when she came to see me, it is necessary to add essential oils to the blend in order to treat the inflammation.

In order to treat Kim, I added three drops of **chamomile** oil, five drops of **tea** tree oil, five drops of **lavender** oil, and five drops of **achillea** oil to the blend. (We can choose each one of the following essential oils and include it in the blend: **peppermint, chamomile, achillea, lavender,** and **tea tree.**) When the condition is not inflamed, we can choose any one of the essential oils in the list above as suitable for treating psoriasis, as long as we use no more than a total of 20 drops of essential oil in the blend of carrier oils.

Kim underwent a general massage once a week, using the blend I prepared for her, in order to invigorate her body, calm her down, and help eliminate the toxins and restore the natural balance of the body. She received a bottle with the same blend to take home, so that she could apply it to the psoriatic areas twice a day, morning and evening. In addition, I prepared a bottle of neat essential oils for Kim, containing **chamomile, lavender, tea tree,** and **achillea** oils in equal quantities. I asked her to drip five to six drops of this blend into a warm bath, and lie in the bath for about 15 to 20 minutes, twice a week. Moreover, I asked her to use the blend in an oil burner during the day, dripping 10 to 12 drops of the pure essential oil into the saucer of the burner, and letting the fragrance fill the room.

After the first two weeks of treatment, Kim did not see much difference in the appearance of the psoriatic areas, but from the point of view of movement, there was a slight difference. She felt that it was easier to move her elbows than usual, but did not feel a great difference in her knees. The massage gave her a very liberating and pleasant feeling, and energized her. She mentioned that the daily massage (she did it twice a day, morning and evening), prevented the skin on her knees and elbows from cracking, which sometimes happened during an outbreak of the disease, and had sometimes even reached the point of infection. For a few hours after the massage, the movement in her elbows was much easier, but after a time, it returned to more or less its previous condition.

We continued the treatment for three months (in which there were ups and downs in the results of the treatment), and gradually Kim reported that she was seeing a substantial improvement in the condition of the psoriatic areas. The skin on her elbows and knees began to be less hard and dry, and a little more soft and pliant, and the formation of scales began to be slower, whereas in the past they had formed a thicker layer. Kim felt a substantial and significant relief in the itching and the pain of the psoriatic areas. The itching disappeared almost totally, and the pain became much less and almost imperceptible.

One of the treatment's more significant successes concerned the inflamed state of the disease. When Kim first came for treatment, there were vesicles full of white pus in certain parts of the psoriatic areas. After persisting with the treatment, most of the vesicles disappeared.

Kim continued with the self-treatment for a long time, since she felt a great improvement in the movement of her elbows and knees, as well as in the esthetic aspect of the disease. During the treatment, we changed the blend of essential oils several times, switching one or more oils each time.

During the same period, Kim also began holistic treatment that included healing and positive thinking, and this helped her accept herself as she was without being ashamed of the disease. During the treatment, she realized how much energy she had wasted on shame and on being afraid of "what people will think and what people will say," energy that she could have kept for herself and directed toward enrichment and positive channels. This treatment gave her the most significant emotional relief, and it may have played a big role in her progress toward healing the disease.

After a time, the disease went into remission. When it appeared again, it was far less severe than in its previous occurrences, and the outbreak was much shorter.

Despite the significant improvement, Kim continued to treat the psoriatic areas on a daily basis, and continued the holistic and macrobiotic treatments in order to maintain the results that had been achieved, as well as to improve her condition.

Dermatitis

Early one morning, my neighbor's son, Mitch, knocked on the door of my clinic. He was suffering from a serious skin infection on his right forearm. Since he had undergone several aromatherapy treatments for similar problems in the past, he decided to come and see whether aromatherapy could help him. Mitch worked in a fiberglass plant, and the day before, he had come into contact with one of the chemicals. He had not been burned, but he began to feel an annoying and bothersome itch. Gradually, the skin of his arm had become red and swollen, very itchy and burning. At first, he had applied a bit of talc to the area, but this did not help very much.

The problem Mitch was suffering from was dermatitis. Dermatitis is a severe skin infection that occurs in the majority of cases as a result of harmful external factors such as chemicals, heat, cold, the sun's rays and other forms of radiation – and is usually located in the affected area only. Dermatitis can be identified according to the following signs: the skin becomes red and swollen, the affected area is itchy, a burning and hot sensation is felt there, as well as a possible wetness, vesicles appear, and there are scabs or scaliness. In these cases, the first thing to do is to avoid the cause of the infection. In mild cases, it is enough to sprinkle a bit of talc on the area. In more severe cases, ointments are prescribed by physicians – and sometimes these ointments contain cortisone. However, treatment with aromatherapy is very effective in various cases of dermatitis.

When treating dermatitis, we must use oils that soothe the skin, treat the itching and burning, and help the skin heal and regenerate itself. Moreover, we must see that we use oils with an analgesic action on the nerve endings, and carrier oils with many minerals and vitamins.

In order to prepare a blend for Mitch to apply locally, I chose the following oils: **melissa**, which is very effective in calming an allergic reaction in the skin and in relieving inflamed swelling; **cedarwood**, which, among other things, helps treat the itching in red, inflamed skin, and disinfects and soothes the skin; **juniper**, which is marvelous in general for skin problems, helps strengthen the skin, and serves as an effective disinfectant and skin cleanser; it also promotes the rapid knitting and healing of tissues and is an effective regenerator; and **cajeput**, which is a superb analgesic.

As a carrier oil, I chose to use **grapeseed** oil, which is absorbed in the body easily, shrinks and knits tissues, and is good for a whole range of problems that stem from sensitive skin, allergies, and rashes. I used 20 cc of **grapeseed** oil in the blend, and added 5 cc of **evening primrose** oil, which helps prevent processes of inflammation and allergies in the body. In addition, I added 5 cc of **olive** oil, because of its analgesic properties, and its effectiveness in cases of skin infections. To the blend of carrier oils I added four drops of **cajeput** oil, five drops of **melissa** oil, four drops of **cedarwood** oil, and two drops of **juniper** oil.

I asked Mitch to apply the blend to the affected area at least three times a day, or every time he felt an itching, a prickling, or an unpleasant sensation there.

Mitch applied the blend and was happy to tell me, two days later, that the redness and swelling had disappeared almost entirely, and the itching had decreased significantly, as had the burning sensation.

A day later, he felt almost no discomfort in his arm at all.

In more serious cases, or when the client does not come for treatment immediately (four or more days after the onset of the infection), a longer time might be required in order to cure the infection. Moreover, in cases in which a person suffers from dermatitis several times a year, he has to check whether it is an allergic reaction to some substance, and whether he has to reinforce his immune system as a significant part of the treatment.

Acne

Acne is one of the most common skin diseases. It occurs in 85% of adolescents, and, in most cases, passes by age 20. (However, there are adults who suffer from the disease, and it can occur at any age.) Frequently, the disease is a result of a hormonal imbalance.

Acne is an annoying and irksome disease, and when it reaches serious proportions that spoil the adolescent's external appearance, it sometimes causes his/her self-esteem to plummet. As I said before, acne can occur at different stages in life. In infants, it can appear as a result of an innate hormonal imbalance, or it can be transferred to them via their mother, and then spots appear on their faces. Adolescent acne is often linked to hormone levels, and can occasionally begin as early as age 10 or 11, depending on personal development. Acne can also occur at ages 20 to 30 as a result of a hormonal condition, a harsh diet, pregnancy, and sometimes even emotional factors. There are women who suffered from acne and recovered from it during pregnancy; in contrast, there are women whose acne occurred during pregnancy. Acne can occur during menopause. Menopausal acne is generally caused by changes in the hormonal balance, poor nutrition, and so on. Additional factors that are thought to be involved in the process of acne formation are allergies, problems of digestion and absorption of fats and carbohydrates, intolerance of dairy products, relative overeating of saturated fats, and so on. Acne occurs mainly in areas of the body that are rich in sebaceous glands, such as the face, the back, the chest, and the shoulders.

Acne can be divided into two forms: non-inflamed acne and inflamed acne.

Non-inflamed acne is less serious, both from the point of view of treatment and from the point of view of coping socially, since it does not entail infected sores. In this type of acne, there are sores that are called comedones. There are two types of comedones: open black ones, that is, there is a partial blockage of the hair by the abnormal keratin that is produced by the skin cells (the keratin is produced by the keratinocyte cell that is located on the innermost layer of the skin, the epidermis. The keratinocyte cell produces a protein that is called keratin, and this protein fills the cytoplasm of the epidermal cells), but air can still pass back and forth to the inside of the skin, causing the sebum to oxidize and become black. That is when we notice blackheads on the skin. The second type of comedones are the closed white ones. Here, the hair that comes out of the skin is completely blocked by the keratin, so the sebum cannot oxidize (because oxygen cannot pass back and forth), and a whitehead is formed. In general, the sores (especially the black comedones) spread over the nose, the forehead, the cheeks, and the chin, and may sometimes spread over the entire face in varying degrees of severity.

Inflamed acne is not esthetic, and can also be detrimental to the facial skin in the long run. The comedones become infected sores called cysts or nodules that are likely to leave scars after healing and for this reason must be treated. There are conditions in which they occur on a one-time basis, such as before a period or as a result of stress or certain foods, such as chocolate or nuts. It is important to take note of when they appear and the environmental circumstances that caused them. When the acne is severe, with cysts on the skin and bacteria-filled abscesses, and there is a serious infection that reaches the point of bleeding, the person must take antibiotics.

Amy, an 18-year-old girl, came for treatment with aromatherapy because of the inflamed acne that had plagued her for many years. Her acne began in a light, non-inflamed form when she first got her period at age 12, and Amy did not pay special attention to it, since the majority of the girls and boys in her class had begun to show similar signs. However, her condition soon developed into inflamed acne, and then Amy began to seek treatment. For three years, she took antibiotics. Antibiotic medications used for treating acne, are very powerful and kill the bacteria. In Amy's case, the medications helped only part of the time, and caused a serious yeast infection that forced her to stop using them. The constant use of antibiotics caused the yeast infection, candida, to develop in her body. (It is important to know that many cases of candida stem from prolonged use of antibiotics, including the type of antibiotic used for treating acne! For this reason, it is very important, when using these medications, that the physician prescribe a concomitant supplementary anti-candida treatment.) After that, she was treated with a medication that is a bi-product of vitamin A and is administered in tablet form, and is used only in cases of inflamed acne. While this medication was found to be effective, and even prevented acne scars, it caused side effects such as dryness in Amy's lips and face, and a rise in her sugar level that lasted as long as she took the tablets.

Amy felt that the treatment with medications was not beneficial for her and caused her great discomfort. At this point, she was in college, and was suffering from ongoing low self-esteem because of the condition of her face, which was covered in inflamed pimples and scabs. Amy's skin was very sensitive, red, and inflamed. Moreover, she mentioned that her acne condition sometimes worsened before her period. Amy described her inner feelings toward herself as a result of the acne, and told me that she tended to become stressed out easily and that she was very shy and hypersensitive, and often felt miserable.

The best treatment for Amy included elements over and above aromatherapy treatment. In Amy's case, it was suggested that she undergo nutritional and orthomolecular balancing (with food supplements, vitamins, and minerals) and treatment with Bach flowers and healing, since it was impossible to ignore the emotional scars and her low self-esteem, and these had to be treated inclusively and holistically.

Aromatherapy for acne is extremely effective. There are many success stories, but, when preparing the blend, it is important to match the oils very carefully to the client himself, and to the circumstances of the occurrence of their acne.

To this end, it must be remembered first and foremost that acne stems from a combination of three factors: over-secretion of sebum, secretion of abnormally structured keratin, and the thriving of three bacteria that are found in the hair follicles of everyone and inside the hairs that come out of the skin. Moreover, there may be hormonal causes that promote the development of acne in the particular person.

Taking into account that in the occurrence of acne, there is a change in the level of secretion from the sebaceous glands or in the viscosity of the secretion, it is important to ensure that the face is clean in order not to encourage sebum accumulation. It is important that the waste all comes out and does not create blockages. The pores fill up and comedones are liable to form as a result of the oxidation of the fats that are present in the sebum. The body interprets this secretion as a foreign element and stimulates a counter-reaction that ultimately exacerbates the situation – a pimple.

The oils used for treating acne are antibiotic and anti-inflammatory, oils that promote and improve circulation, oils that help purify and disinfect, oils that balance sebum secretion, oils for soothing inflamed skin, and, of course, any additional oils that may be needed according to the nature of the client's complaints.

The oils that are recommended for the treatment of acne are **tea tree, lavender, lemon, sandalwood, bergamot, chamomile, geranium,** and **melissa** (and there are many more). **Eucalyptus** is also frequently used, since in addition to being a good stimulator of circulation, it is also a powerful disinfectant. **Clary sage** and **ylang ylang** are oils that balance sebum, and are therefore suitable for inclusion in the blend for treating acne.

For Amy's treatment, I chose the following oils: **lemon**, which is a powerful disinfectant, astringent, antiseptic, antibacterial, and, in addition, is effective in lightening blotches and scars and in promoting skin tone. In addition, **lemon** oil helps reinforce the immune system and promote leukocyte production.

Reinforcing the immune system is a criterion that is stressed when preparing an aromatic blend, because it is important to include an oil that reinforces the immune system at a certain stage in every blend. This is very important in the case of acne, where various allergic factors are sometimes involved. **Lavender** oil, which is antiseptic, antibacterial, soothes inflammations, and soothes the skin in general, helps lighten blotches and scars and creates an even appearance. It is suitable for red, inflamed skin, promotes regeneration – the renewal of cells and tissues – and also reinforces the immune system. We must not ignore the effective work of **lavender** in the emotional realm. It is calming and creates a very pleasant feeling, which was very important in Amy's case.

The additional oil I chose was **chamomile**. I chose it because of its powerful anti-inflammatory properties, its effectiveness in cases of severe acne, its suitability for inflamed, red, and sensitive skin, and, of course, for its superb work from the emotional point of view. It is an essential oil that helps in cases of stress, pressure, and a need to calm down, hypersensitivity, and even cases of tension and depression as a result of hormonal imbalance (which was likely to be the case with Amy).

The last oil I chose was **clary sage**, which is used in aromatherapy treatment of acne because it balances hormonal action, improves and promotes circulation, and balances sebum secretion.

I prepared two blends from these oils. The first, which was pure, without any carrier oils, was to be used in Amy's baths and facial compresses. The second, which contained carrier oil, was to be used for massage.

The primary treatment for acne, in this case, was the compress. There are various cosmetic treatments that tend to be more powerful and concentrated, but they can only be administered by professional aromatherapist-beauticians. The treatment described below, in contrast, is gentle, and can be administered at home.

The first blend, the neat one, was prepared in a 10-cc bottle. I added 20 drops of **clary sage** oil, 10 crops of **chamomile** oil, 15 drops of **lemon** oil, and 20 drops of **lavender** oil. Again, it is important to remember, especially in a case in which we prepare a pure blend, that several drops of each oil must be placed alternately in the bottle and balanced according to their smell, since different makes of oil are liable to be of different strengths. Since the blend contains **lemon** oil, which is a phototoxic oil, the client must not be exposed to the sun for 12 hours after the application of the oil. For this reason, I asked Amy to perform all the treatments that she had to do at home in the evening, before going to sleep. As a rule, baths and compresses (mainly cosmetic compresses) should be done before resting or going to sleep, since this provides the body with the time and relaxation necessary for making the most of the properties of the oil.

The compress is prepared by dripping five drops of the pure blend into a quart of warm water. I asked Amy to soak a clean white cotton cloth in this mixture and to cover her face with it for half an hour. (In this case, the length of time for the compress was increased, as was the number of drops of oil in the water, for two reasons. First, the serious infected state of Amy's face, and second, the oils we used for treating this particular case were mainly delicate oils with a low level of toxicity – the **lavender**, the **chamomile**, and the **clary sage**). In general, it is advisable to follow the regular instructions for preparing a compress, unless the therapist has a great deal of knowledge of and experience in aromatherapy.

During the first week, Amy was to apply compresses to her face three times a day, the first time for a half-hour, and the other two times for 15 minutes each. During the second week, she was to apply the compresses twice a day for 20 minutes each time. After that, she could reduce the frequency to three times a week, once or twice each day, according to her progress and personal feeling. (I reminded her to avoid being in the sunlight during this time because of the phototoxicity of the **lemon** oil in the blend.)

Moreover, Amy was to take an aromatic bath three times during the first week. This was very important, both for helping her general condition, and also because of the fact that various parts of her body (her shoulders, back, and buttocks) were not free of acne, even though the state of the acne in those places was not nearly as serious, and it was not inflamed. While she was in the bath, she was to relax, preferably with the help of pleasant, quiet music, do abdominal breathing exercises, and let her body heal and the essential oils do their work. After the bath, she was not to soap herself or take a shower. She was to dry herself off gently so that the essential oils remained on her body for as long as possible.

When treating acne, it is important to treat the whole body in parallel to the treatment with facial compresses, in order to stimulate it to excrete waste and reinforce itself. For this reason, it is worthwhile including whole-body massage in the treatment. We performed this massage twice during the first week, and once a week for the subsequent month. I prepared the massage blend from 20 cc of **apricot kernel** oil, 10 cc of **sunflower** oil (cold pressed), nine drops of **lavender** oil, five drops of **chamomile** oil, six drops of **lemon** oil, and six drops of **clary sage** oil. (Note: the amount of essential oil in the blend is larger than usual!)

After two weeks of massages, compresses, baths, and heating the pure oil blend in an oil burner with water, Amy felt some relief in her condition. Now we moved on to the "cosmetic" stage of the treatment, which was performed in parallel to the home treatment with compresses and baths and in parallel to the massage.

The cosmetic-aromatherapy treatment suggested for acne is very effective, but must only be administered by a qualified cosmetician. First of all, we cleansed Amy's face with special cosmetic soap that suited her skin. Then we prepared a facial mask with gel. Two drops of **lemon** oil were added to the gel because of its superb disinfectant properties. After spreading the gel on Amy's face, we placed gauze on the gel layer and on them we placed a compress made of a felt mask soaked in rose water. (To prepare the compress, we used two drops of **rosewater** in two cups of water.) We covered the felt mask with plastic wrap (leaving openings for the nose and mouth, of course) and left it on for about 10 minutes. The cosmetician gradually exposed bit after bit of Amy's face while she worked at removing the comedones. When she had finished removing the comedones and the mask, the beautician disinfected Amy's face with skin tonic that was suitable for her skin. Then another mask was placed on Amy's face, for soothing the skin, for balancing it, and for treating the acne scars. This mask was prepared from a teaspoonful of neutral gel to which a teaspoon of **apricot kernel** oil, two drops of **peppermint** oil, and two drops of **lavender** oil were added. The cosmetician spread the blend over Amy's face, and, about 10 minutes later, washed it off with warm water.

After the cosmetic treatment, there was a significant improvement in Amy's facial skin. It looked cleaner of acne since many of the comedones had been extracted, its color had improved, and it looked lighter and glowed.

Now, all Amy had to do was to continue the home treatment with compresses and massage, and carry on with the holistic treatment. After three months of treatment, during which Amy had another cosmetic-aromatherapy treatment for her acne, there was an obvious improvement in the condition of her face. Now, she only had a few inflamed pimples left on her face; most of the infected pimples had disappeared. The acne on her body disappeared almost totally. Her facial skin looked cleaner (beforehand, her skin had looked flawed, scarred, and blotchy), and the areas where the acne spread were significantly reduced. Now, in order to continue the healing process, until the problem was completely eliminated, Amy would have to continue applying the compresses once or twice a week, take at least one bath a week, and continue with her holistic treatment and her nutritional balancing. She was delighted with the improvement in her condition, and besides the significant improvement in the acne problem, she also felt a substantial change in her mood and in her general feeling.

Athlete's foot

Brian, a 19-year-old football player, arrived with a problem that had begun six months previously. In the past, he had suffered from athlete's foot several times, and now it seemed as if he had been infected during training once again. His condition was bothering him particularly badly. The fungal infection was located between his toes, was very itchy, and really bothered him during training. He also suffered from fungal infections on his toenails, which, although they did not itch, distorted the shape of the nails and made them thick and yellow.

Although he was not overly worried about the fungal infections, he realized that it was essential for him to treat them immediately, because they bothered him, and they could get worse.

A fungal infection on the foot is caused by a fungus that settles between the toes. Its "favorite" place is generally between the two small toes. A place that is infected with a fungus displays red marks, peeling, a dry and scaly rash on the skin or between the toes, and an annoying itch.

The fungus can spread over the foot and toenails, which thicken and become yellow as a result.

Many people who suffer from this disease do not treat it properly, and for this reason may well suffer from it for a long time. There are people who live with fungal infections on their feet for their entire lives when it is actually possible to solve the problem with a simple but lasting treatment.

Fungal infections can be contracted in public showers, locker rooms, sports and recreation centers, on hikes, and in the military, so when using public showers, it is extremely important to wear rubber shoes and not to use someone else's towel. In addition, it is important to air the feet, especially after walking or wearing a closed shoe for a long time, and to see that the feet are clean and dry, since the fungus thrives in warm, moist, and dark places.

Of course, it is important to keep the bathroom clean and disinfected, and when a member of the household suffers from a fungal infection on the foot, the shower and bathroom should be cleaned with bleach in order to prevent the rest of the family from becoming infected.

The treatment of fungal infections on the feet is very simple and enjoys a very high success rate. The blend I prepared for Brian contained 30 cc of **wheatgerm** oil, to which I added 10 drops of **tea tree** oil, which is an extremely powerful disinfectant, and possesses treatment properties that are very effective in cases of fungi and bacteria, 10 drops of **lavender** oil, and five drops of **lemon** oil, which is a very powerful antibacterial and disinfectant oil. (Note: The proportion of essential oils to carrier oil is higher than usual.)

I asked Brian to apply the blend to the skin around his toenails three times a day, and to apply pure **lavender** oil between his toes twice a day.

Brian tried the treatment for a few days and experienced immediate relief. After persisting with the treatment, and applying the blend to the skin around his toenails, as well as applying **lavender** oil between his toes, the fungal infections became a thing of the past, and all Brian had to do was to ensure hygienic conditions for his feet so that he would not be infected again.

Although there were almost no more signs of the fungal infection after a long period of treatment, I suggested that Brian administer a "maintenance" dose once a week in order to preserve the status quo.

Dandruff

Nadine, a 35-year-old lawyer, had suffered from an annoying dandruff problem for many years. As an impressive and well-groomed woman, this problem bothered her enormously. She spent a lot of time on skin and hair care, used various anti-dandruff shampoos and cosmetics, and had become a veritable expert on the subject. Occasionally, the shampoos helped solve the problem, but when she stopped using them and resorted to a regular shampoo, the problem returned, and her hair became full of white flakes of dandruff.

Dandruff consists of dead cells that peel off the skin of the scalp. They are silvery-white in color, and can be seen on the hair, the collar and shoulders, and, in serious cases, on the back of the clothing. Dandruff is a very common problem (about 30% of the population suffers from it), and it is more common among people with oily skin. It does not constitute any kind of physical problem, but can mar the esthetic look of the hair.

The causes of dandruff are not yet known, but it is possible that, like balding, it stems from emotional causes such as tension, pressure, and aggravation; from hormonal imbalance; or from allergies and sensitivity to various substances.

Many essential oils are used in the symptomatic treatment of dandruff, as are various types of shampoo that are available. Among the essential oils that are suitable for treating dandruff are **patchouli, cedarwood**, and **rosemary**. For a more in-depth treatment, it is a good idea to check whether the person displays other signs of hormonal imbalance (these could be hairiness, acne and frequent pimples on the skin, menstrual irregularity, and so on), whether he is allergic or sensitive to various substances, and whether he is exposed to constant tension and stress as a result of his work and lifestyle or his personality type.

Aromatherapy treatment for dandruff includes one or two of the following oils: **patchouli, cedarwood**, or **rosemary**. Altogether four drops of the essential oil/s are added to 10 cc of **jojoba** carrier oil. The blend is used to perform a deep and long massage of the scalp, and afterwards, the oil is left on the head for a half-hour to two hours. After the treatment, the hair should be washed with a shampoo meant for daily use, to which a few drops of **patchouli** or **tea tree** oils have been added. This treatment is effective in most cases of dandruff, and it should be repeated as needed. These oils can be used when adding oils that treat the cause of the problem, if it can be defined.

After a long interview, it turned out that Nadine was exposed to constant pressure and stress in her work. Her daily schedule was exacting and crowded, and she was highly achievement-oriented, as well as being a perfectionist. Success in court was of tremendous importance to her. She worked under a great deal of pressure for long hours, sometimes 10 or 12 hours a day, and there were long periods in which she was swamped with work, and only devoted a little time to relaxing and releasing tension. Moreover, she suffered from inner agitation that grew as the pressure of work increased and she had a deadline to meet, or before an appearance in court. Sometimes, she would feel slightly anxious (quite naturally) before appearing in court, but she would ignore the feeling and go on as usual.

When I asked Nadine when she had first started suffering from dandruff, she mentioned the beginning of her career as the starting point of the problem. Because of those findings, it is possible that the tension and pressure she was under played an important and influential role in the onset of the problem and its exacerbation.

In order to make the treatment more effective, I decided to add **clary sage** oil to the blend. In Nadine's case, it would help treat two additional aspects: the first was her greasy scalp (a common condition in people who have dandruff), and the second was the agitation, tension, and anxiety that **clary sage** helps calm down to a large extent. Moreover, I included **patchouli** oil in the blend, because, besides its contribution to the treatment of dandruff, it also soothes and alleviates states of tension and stress.

Ultimately, I prepared a blend from 10 cc of **jojoba** carrier oil, two drops of **cedarwood** oil, one drop of **patchouli** oil, and one drop of **clary sage** oil.

Another way of preparing the blend is by using two drops each of **cedarwood** and **patchouli** oils only.

Nadine administered the treatment once a week. After doing so, her hair was soft and shiny, and almost totally free of dandruff. She continued with the treatment regularly, and gradually noticed that she needed it less frequently. She enjoyed both the esthetic success of the treatment and the wonderful soothing properties of the oils.

Emotional problems

Since ancient times, essential oils have been used to treat emotional states, from honing the ability to concentrate, think, and learn, treating depression, agitation, insomnia, hysteria and so on, to serving as aphrodisiacs for promoting sexual arousal and fanning the flames of passion.

The field of psycho-aromatherapy is being studied in research laboratories in many universities throughout the world. In the past, experiments with essential oils were performed on mental patients, and today there are various centers in the world that focus on the study of the effect of aromatic fragrances on emotional and physiological conditions. Many attempts are being made to introduce the use of essential oils into hospitals using either massage or oil burners.

There are hospitals throughout the world that use aromatic fragrances in the reception rooms of terminal wards in order to create a soothing and calming atmosphere for the family when they are given bad news about the condition of their loved one. Other experiments are being conducted in psychiatric centers with patients who are given large doses of sleeping pills and tranquilizers. When the oils are used over time, it was found that the patients' dosage of medications could be decreased. In these cases, the main oil used was **lavender** because of its psychological and physical effects. In studies involving high-school students suffering from memory and concentration problems, it was found that after a few months of treatment with suitable essential oils for improving memory and concentration, there was an improvement in their ability to concentrate, study, and remember the material.

The action of the oils on people's emotional states is surprising in its intensity. It is easier to understand how the process works when we look at how the sense of smell and the different areas of the brain react to the oils. The sense of smell is a chemical sense, as is the sense of taste, and it also reacts to chemical energy (as opposed to other senses that react to "waves" of mechanical energy). It was found that the sense of smell reacted best to the essential oils.

In each nostril, there are nerve cells – neurons that end in many dendrites, each of which terminates in a so-called bulb, which is the specific receptor for the molecules of the odor. The axons of the neurons comprise the olfactory nerve that is located in the nostrils and goes to the brain where it reaches the central lobe – the limbic lobe. The limbic lobe is the seat of the emotions, memories, sexual feelings, learning, and so on. The odor itself reaches the brain and the limbic lobe in two ways: by passing through the membranes and the "barrier" of the brain, and via an electric pulse that creates a potential for action. For this reason, the beginning of the emotional effect as a result of odor occurs only after a few seconds.

The intensity and effect of the odor on the body and the brain is emphasized by the fact that only a few molecules of the odor are sufficient to stimulate many receptors to action, and only the smallest amount is required to feel the difference.

Having said that, the rapid adaptation to odor must be taken into consideration, since because of it, we can smell over and over again. This adaptation has three causes: the many floods of saliva that cause the smell molecules to dissolve; a prolonged and powerful action on the central nervous system, which causes a decline in the ability to smell for a short time (after a brief rest, it is once again possible to smell at the same intensity. Part of the adaptation reaction to smells is attributed to the body's defense mechanism); in addition, during exhalation, we expel air (and this "eliminates" the molecules of odor).

And there are still molecules of odor that succeed in going up to the brain, since the barrier is not hermetic, and they enter the limbic lobe and have an effect.

In order to understand how the essential oils affect many forms of behavior and a broad range of emotional and nervous sensations, we must look at the limbic lobe and the glands located in it, which have many rational-emotional functions.

The limbic lobe is located deep in the brain, between the thalamus and the cortex. The brainstem is also located in the vicinity of the limbic lobe, and it is considered to be part of the limbic system. Its function is to transmit messages from the system to the body and from the body to the system. Through this system of transmitting messages, sexual desires, the survival instinct, and so on, are expressed and experienced.

There are many glands that are responsible for a range of functions in the limbic system:

The *thalamus*, a large gland that serves as a transmitting station for information connected with feeling and movement, processes the data and transmits them to the cortex (the outer layer of the brain). All sensory information that reaches the skin is linked to the thalamus.

Below the thalamus is the *hypothalamus*, whose function is to receive messages and transfer them to the brainstem, via the thalamus, and to the pituitary gland, in order to activate hormone-secreting glands. Moreover, it is responsible for maintaining the stability of the internal environment, and for maintaining the will to live, so it has a very powerful behavioral and emotional effect (conditions of thirst as well as stimuli linked to anger, fear, sexual behavior, or aggressiveness stem from the hypothalamus).

Another gland is the *amygdala*, whose principal action takes place on the emotional and behavioral plane, on the subconscious level, through which the person receives a report about his condition vis-à-vis his surroundings, and interprets his condition in a behavioral manner. When the amygdala of lab monkeys was extracted, there were changes in the animals' eating habits and way of processing the sensation of fear, a decrease in aggressiveness, and an increase in their sexual urge.

Below the temporal lobe is the *hippocampus*, whose function is to pick up information and decisions and send them to the memory. It is connected with learning and memory. This area is also linked to epilepsy, so an overly-powerful stimulation can cause an electrical short circuit in the brain and an epileptic seizure (from this we understand the action of oils that may cause an epileptic seizure).

There is another gland that is linked to the pain phenomenon in general and the alleviation of pain in particular, and contains neurons that secrete neurotransmitters, among them serotonin. When serotonin is secreted, it causes a general calming down and relaxing of muscles. The effect of the oils on this gland causes the secretion of serotonin, thereby increasing the calming and relaxing effect. Serotonin prevents the contraction of blood vessels, prevents depression, and has a soothing, relaxing, and hypnotic effect. It plays an important role in the action of the brain and the nervous system as well as in normal intestinal action (large amounts of alcohol and tranquilizers damage this secretion). The sleep mechanism also depends on this gland.

Another important gland is the *pituitary*, which is located at the front of the pineal gland, and serves as a kind of control center that regulates many functions. It is indirectly linked to the limbic system by secreting hormones that are also linked to balanced behavior and emotions. It consists of two lobes, each with its own character, and each secreting different kinds of hormones:

Tropic hormones – these are hormones that are secreted by one endocrine gland and activate another endocrine gland – for instance, the sex hormones FSH or TSH.

Somatic hormones – these are hormones that are secreted by endocrine glands and directly affect the body's cells – for instance, the growth hormone, the anti-diuretic hormone, and so on.

The various decisions are made in the limbic system, pass through the cortex, via the motor nervous system and via the autonomic system (to the internal organs), and cause the secretion of neurotransmitters and hormones for activating the body in a balanced manner between body and mind.

From this we can understand the importance of the use of the oil burner and its significant effect on body and mind alike.

It is possible to discern the actions of the different types of oils on different areas of the brain – the soothing oils affect the secretion of serotonin. The mentally stimulating oils affect the hippocampus and the amygdala. The aphrodisiac oils affect the pituitary via the hypothalamus. The euphoria-inducing oils affect the hypothalamus, and the analgesic oils affect the hypothalamus and the pituitary.

When we look at the essential oils that are used for treating emotional problems, we find that for almost every emotional disturbance or imbalance there are essential oils that can help balance the problem.

The oils must be divided up into the following categories: soothing oils, invigorating oils, stimulating oils, and emotionally balancing oils. Certain oils possess several properties, even properties that seem to be contradictory, such as **marjoram**, which is both soothing and invigorating, or **peppermint**, which is soothing and sleep-inducing in a large quantity, and stimulating in a small quantity. There are also other subcategories.

Among the soothing oils are the following: **grapefruit, bergamot, lavender** (it must be remembered that **lavender** oil "adapts" itself to the general blend, and reinforces it. In a soothing blend, it fortifies the soothing effect, and in an invigorating blend, it can reinforce the invigorating effect a little), **oregano, ylang ylang, benzoin, angelica, Siberian fir, lemon, marjoram, melissa, mandarine, neroli, cedarwood, sandalwood, petitgrain, patchouli, clary sage, chamomile, rosewood, frankincense, lemongrass, parsley, jasmine, louisa, myrrh, laurel, rose, rosewater, vetiver, marigold** (which is also stimulating), **tangerine, dill** and **orange** (all the citrus oils have a soothing effect).

Among the invigorating oils are the following: **marjoram** (which, as we said before, is both invigorating and soothing), **eucalyptus, fennel, angelica, basil,**

juniper, **lemon** (also soothing), **peppermint** (which is soothing in large quantities), **niaouli**, **sage**, **cajeput**, **camphor**, **chamomile** (which is also very soothing), **rosemary** and **thyme**.

Among the stimulating oils are the following: **peppermint** (when used in small quantities), **cajeput**, **patchouli**, **petitgrain**, **sage**, **nutmeg**, **achillea**, **eucalyptus**, **cedarwood**, **grapefruit** (also soothing), **bergamot** (also soothing), **wintergreen**, **ginger**, **everlasting**, **galbanum**, **coriander**, **frankincense** (also soothing), **lemon** (also soothing and invigorating), **mandarine**, **marigold** (also soothing), **niaouli**, **spearmint**, **juniper**, **black pepper**, **citronella**, **clove**, **red thyme**, **caraway**, **cinnamon**, **camphor**, **cardamon**, and **rosemary**.

The analgesic oils are: **galbanum**, **lavender**, **birch**, **sage**, **niaouli**, **celery**, **laurel**, **black pepper**, **chamomile**, **rosewood**, and **rosemary**.

Among the oils that help bring about emotional equilibrium are the following: **grapefruit**, **cedarwood**, **clary sage**, **cypress**, **niaouli**, **lavender**, **tea tree**, **yarrow**, **patchouli**, **juniper**, **geranium**, **melissa**, **lemon**, and **orange**.

There are numerous anti-depressant oils. Among them are: **grapefruit**, **neroli**, **sandalwood**, **chamomile**, **clary sage** (which causes a pleasantly euphoric feeling), **patchouli**, **rose**, and **mandarine**. **Petitgrain** is also a light anti-depressant, and **vetiver** helps in conditions in which depression results from a lack or drop in the estrogen level in the body.

Certain oils, which can give a feeling of jubilation, are called "uplifting" oils. Their fragrance causes an improvement in mood, sometimes even of joy and gaiety. Among these oils are **bergamot**, **melissa**, **petitgrain**, **basil**, and **rosewood**. **Clary sage** oil causes a euphoric feeling, and is not recommended for use prior to driving. **Rose**, **melissa**, and **marjoram** help a great deal in conditions of melancholy and sorrow.

Conditions of hysteria, too, can be relieved by sniffing or using essential oils. **Lavender**, **neroli**, **clary sage**, **frankincense**, **camphor**, **melissa**, **orange**, **chamomile**, and **peppermint** can be very helpful in these conditions, in conjunction, of course, with proper psychological treatment, when the condition is frequent and disrupts the person's normal functioning.

Clary sage, **frankincense**, and **melissa** are recommended for treating states of panic. In this context, it must be mentioned that when treating emotional problems, aromatherapy is performed on people suffering from an *emotional imbalance*, and not on people who are defined as chronic or temporary sufferers from a mental disturbance. In these cases, aromatherapy has a great and important effect, but the treatment must be administered by a qualified professional aromatherapist, in conjunction with the other conventional or supplementary treatment the client is receiving. People who are mentally ill must not be treated with essential oils without professional knowledge and experience, especially because the oils have such an obvious and powerful effect in the treatment of mental problems.

The use of oils is recommended in cases of mourning, loss, or separation as well (the easiest way is, of course, the use of an oil burner, which, in states of emotional imbalance, is extremely effective). In such cases, **rose** and **melissa** oil can be an excellent choice.

In cases of a feeling of loneliness and alienation, the use of **marjoram** or **mandarine** oil can alleviate the condition. These oils are also used to treat cases of various traumas. **Frankincense** and **benzoin** are known to cause a feeling of protection and safety from external factors, and **juniper** oil helps in cases involving a feeling of dirt and impurity. (It must be remembered that in professional treatment, the emphasis will be placed on understanding the reasons for these feelings and the treatment of those reasons together with soothing the emotional symptoms.) The essential oil helps restore a feeling of cleanliness and purity.

When we treat a physical problem, and also discover that the client suffers a great deal from anger, irritation, and resentment, it is a good idea to add one of the following oils to the blend: **vetiver, grapefruit, chamomile**, or **mandarine**.

In states of hypersensitivity, when the client is very sensitive, easily hurt, easily offended, and tends to see things excessively subjectively, it is advisable to add one of the following oils to the blend: **melissa, chamomile**, or **mandarine**.

For agitation, **lavender, grapefruit, chamomile, orange** and **clary sage** oils can help. When the agitation is accompanied by a headache, **angelica** oil may well be the suitable choice.

A very significant area for which essential oils are used in holistic treatment is for helping to reduce stress and tension. Many practitioners, physicians, and researchers are now reaching the conclusion that one of the many causes of the depletion of the immune system, as well as of interference with overall body functions, is stress.

Stress is a well-known and common concept in the "fast" and achievement-oriented society of today. The daily stresses to which people are subjected are extremely high, and the possibility of finding oneself in states of stress or pressure at work, on the highways, at home – in fact in almost any place – is enormous. Stress is, to all intents and purposes, a physical phenomenon. The emotional process that engenders stress causes the activation of physical mechanisms, and being in states of constant pressure and stress exhausts the body. For many people, situations of not meeting deadlines at work, domestic arguments, pressure in studies, traveling on the highways, financial pressures, and so forth, cause stress and gradually weaken all of the body's systems.

In fact, in one way or another, every holistic treatment touches upon the idea of reducing stress and pressure in order to improve the client's general condition. It is astonishing how much a treatment that helps lower the client's stress level can help him in all areas of life by supporting him mentally and physically, and redirecting the energies that were previously invested in the causes of the stress and in coping with them, to more useful and beneficial purposes. Being in a constant state of stress can exhaust the person physically and mentally and can cause various diseases.

It is well known that there are many diseases that are directly and obviously connected to the client's stress level. Other diseases are substantially exacerbated by states of stress and pressure. Among the diseases that are known to have a strong connection to psychological stress are asthma, various problems in the menstrual cycle, problems in the immune system (exposure to infections and so on), hypertension, ulcers, adult diabetes, arthritis, colitis, headaches and migraines, cancer, heart diseases, circulatory diseases, outbreaks of psoriasis, and so on.

Essential oils effectively and significantly relieve stress. People who are under frequent pressure (this, of course, is a subjective feeling), who are overworked and suffer from a stress-inducing requirement such as deadlines, are advised to make regular use of an oil burner containing a blend of oils that help reduce and relieve states of stress.

Among the oils that are used in a burner are **lavender, vetiver, frankincense, chamomile, rose, neroli,** (especially together with **petitgrain**), **mandarine, cedarwood, ylang ylang, patchouli**, and so on.

Using essential oils, it is also possible to treat mental fatigue and exhaustion, which are often caused by prolonged stress. Generally, **melissa** and **rosewood** oils are known to encourage body and mind. For mental fatigue and exhaustion, it is advisable to use one or more of the following oils: **rosemary, peppermint, marjoram,** and **clary sage**, as well as **pine, lavender** and **neroli**, which treat fatigue and exhaustion via relaxation.

In order to clarify and stimulate thought and memory, it is advisable to use one or more of the following oils: **basil, rosemary, angelica, cinnamon, peppermint**, and **thyme**. These oils also help during stressful periods of studies, and when it is necessary to memorize a great deal of material and remain alert and lucid.

Insomnia can also be treated with essential oils, and the oils that are recommended in this case are **vetiver, ylang ylang, marjoram** (especially in a massage or bath), **lavender, patchouli** (which reduces stress and anxiety), **tangerine**, and **mandarine**. The combination of **neroli** with **petitgrain** also has good results.

Summary

Besides the common problems and the ways of solving them that are described in detail in the book, there are additional emotional problems that can be treated with essential oils. We will try to look deeply into each problem, discover, with the client, the basic causes for it, and treat it using the appropriate essential oil. Of course, we will observe the basic rules – not to use more than four essential oils in the blend, and to administer treatment in accordance with the warnings and counter-indications.

For treating emotional conditions with essential oils, the most effective methods are massage, aromatic baths, the oil burner, and reflexology in combination with essential oils. We must concoct the blend that is suitable for each client's specific problem and his physical and emotional complaints, and create a blend that is holistic and can treat a large number of problems. In many cases, there is an interaction between the client's various physical and emotional problems, and they trigger one another. This causes the problem to remain blocked and unsolved.

It must be remembered and reiterated over and over again that every physical disease has a psychological aspect. Often, the disease is an expression of various mental processes, conscious or unconscious, and as practitioners, we have to know how to identify them, and help free the mind and overcome the emotional obstacles that cause blockages and prevent progress and recovery.

When we treat the emotional side, we help the life energy to flow more easily, thus encouraging the body to heal. It is often possible to find a chain of negative events that cause a disease on the emotional or the physical level, and in most of the cases both of the levels are affected. The chain of negative events may begin from stress or trauma, causing the person to develop a negative attitude toward life. A negative attitude and lack of confidence are an extremely common reason for difficulties in falling asleep and insomnia (amazingly common problems!). When the person finds it difficult to fall asleep because of a high level of pressure, the cumulative fatigue leaves its mark on him. He feels too exhausted to engage in physical activity, and tries to balance the state of fatigue by eating, drinking coffee and using other stimulants. He then begins to feel heavy and listless. When anxiety, depression, existential fears, financial worries or domestic preoccupations are also added to that chain of negative events, the sleeping difficulties increase, and, at the same time, the physiological and immune systems are weakened. The person experiences a bad overall feeling, or tries to compensate for this feeling and for his emotional feelings by smoking, drinking "stimulating" coffee, bingeing, and so on. This state can reach the point of neglect of environmental, physical, and mental hygiene, which, of course, exacerbates the emotional problems even more, and the person is liable to feel a lack of energy at this point. He does not feel like doing things, going out, seeing people, and he locks himself even more into this vicious circle. When we add physical weakness in one of the body's systems, hormonal problems or a hormonal imbalance (especially states of menopause or uncomfortable premenstrual symptoms in women) to the chain of negative events, we get an even heavier "package." In this situation, a disease or problem is liable to occur at a certain point in one of the weaker systems of that person's body. Therefore, many people do not notice the formation of the psycho-physical chain of negative events, and come for treatment only after the disease in one of the body's systems has been felt. When we examine the chain of negative events, we discover pressure, stress, or an emotional or thought imbalance at its beginning. In these cases, our primary target is to return the client to a state of calm and relaxation.

When it comes to restoring relaxation and calmness, the essential oils are truly "magicians," and as we saw at the beginning of the chapter, the range of oils at our disposal for accomplishing this is vast.

In addition, we must not neglect nutritional balance; it is imperative to identify nutritional deficiencies or a defective daily menu, remove unsuitable foods or stimulants (caffeine), and substitute healthy, fortifying foods. Frequently, suitable physical activity is also a necessary or effective aspect of a complete treatment.

When we enable the person to feel calm and relaxed using the range of methods at our disposal in aromatherapy, we enable his body and mind to rest and commence the process of self-balance and accumulation of renewed energy and strength. The renewal of the energy supplies simultaneously leads to better activity during the day, and to a rise in the level of general motivation as well as in the motivation for self-treatment (very important when there is a need for a program of physical exercise, nutritional changes, diet, and so on), and also better and more satisfying sleep. Better sleep promotes the body's self-healing power, and helps change the person's attitude toward his surroundings and bring about a better and calmer general feeling, while reducing the daily level of stress, agitation, and tension. When the person's mood is good, his motivation for balancing his mental and physical state grows and strengthens. This means that he can cope with problems and tasks in a calm, effective, and stress-free way, effect nutritional changes, and do things that are likely to cause him to feel much better and healthier. When the person permits himself the pleasures of life that do him good, eats correctly, and activates his body, he has a healthier and more pliant body and a calmer and more balanced mind. All those, of course, together with a reduction in the level of everyday stress, reinforce his immune system and his body's power of self-healing, and together with the external treatment (that administered by the practitioner) of the disease itself, we significantly increase the chances of a total recovery and the attainment of good health.

Depression

Unfortunately, depression is not in the least uncommon. Many people experience the terrible feeling of depression at least once in their lives – often *as a result of an event that is extreme, traumatic, or painful*. In contrast, there are people who feel down or experience depression *without an obvious, evident reason*, or because of hormonal reasons, changes of season, etc.

Depression is frequently a mental state that is a by-product of a serious disease, or occurs as a result of a break-up, a bad domestic situation, an experience of loss or death, a feeling of failure, being fired from a job, and so on.

In the course of my work as a holistic practitioner, I have encountered this painful problem many times. It can occur in children, teenagers, adults, and the elderly. Sometimes it is a by-product of the change of life in both women and men, of giving birth (post-partum depression), or of the stages of adolescence.

It is not a problem that can be ignored, since it has a significant effect on the person's general state of mind, thoughts, emotions, behavior, and physical condition. The immune system is also greatly affected by a depressed mood, and tends to become drastically weakened in these depressed states.

When treating depression, we must first know how to diagnose it correctly. There are several criteria that can help us diagnose the state and the severity:

Way of thinking: The depressive way of thinking is characterized by seeing "the half-empty glass" – a tendency to see life generally in a pessimistic way, viewing it as tiring, difficult, hopeless, and meaningless. People who have a tendency toward a pessimistic outlook on life are inclined to make incorrect generalizations in their lives. Abandonment by a loved one can be interpreted by these people as a serious blow to their self-esteem, and they make a generalization like: "I'm not worth anything! No one loves me! I will never have a loving partner!" Being fired from a job can be interpreted as personal failure, a feeling of worthlessness, and a tendency to see the failure as a failure in many fields: "I'm nothing, I'm worth nothing, nothing works out for me..." and so on, instead of seeing things in the correct proportion.

"Looking on the dark side" is often accompanied by a feeling of helplessness, by an extreme dissatisfaction with life, and by a feeling that nothing can be done to improve the situation. A depressive state of mind causes the person to view life as a sequence of disappointments and failures, and even positive and pleasant events tend to "disappear" or be forgotten when the person has a profound feeling of a lack of success and ability.

Emotional state: Depression is expressed in its fullest intensity in the emotional realm. The depressive person tends to feel sadness, frustration, tension, anxiety about the present and the future, various fears, and sometimes even anger and rage toward things that did not use to anger him so profoundly. Often, the person feels a decline in his ability to feel positive emotions and derive pleasure from life. Moreover, people who suffer from depression report a feeling of loneliness, boredom and emptiness, as well as a drop in initiative and in the desire and ability to achieve.

Physical state: Physical changes can also be discerned in a state of depression. Depression is often accompanied by crying, fatigue, a lack of energy, and sometimes a feeling of tightness in the chest, nausea, vomiting, headaches, constipation, frequent and constant back and joint pains, and these increase the feeling of depression and suffering.

Sleep: Sleeping a lot is a way of running away from the distressing feeling – and conversely, there can be sleep disruptions such as poor sleep or difficulties in falling asleep. Sometimes, the depressed person tends to wake up in the early hours or finds it difficult to fall asleep until the late hours of the night. Sleep is not continuous and pleasant, either, but rather plagued by disturbing dreams and thoughts. The depressed state also manifests itself in its effect on certain cerebral activities, such as a drop in memory and concentration and a slowness of thought (and sometimes of action, too).

Eating: There can be changes in eating habits, too. The depressive person may suffer from either a lack of appetite or too much appetite and overeating, generally at unlikely hours and irregularly. Depression can be accompanied by either a weight loss or a weight gain.

Sex: The depressed person may suffer from a sharp drop in libido and in the enjoyment of sex, and he is liable to experience difficulties in sexual functioning during the period of depression.

Behavior: Depressive behavior is often characterized by shutting oneself up at home, an unwillingness to see friends or to go out and have a good time, and in a significant decline in the level of activity and functioning. This state is liable to affect the way the person functions as a worker and as a parent, and, in extreme cases, he may even find it difficult to do simple actions such as washing himself, cleaning the home, getting out of bed, going to work, and so on.

As we said before, depression may have many different causes, some of which are listed below:

Physical causes: Physical, hormonal, or biochemical conditions, as well as various diseases, are liable to be expressed in or to cause a feeling of depression. Among the common causes are the use of alcohol, drugs, and medications (these include commonly used medications such as some of those used for treating hypertension and heart problems, and cortisone).

Hormonal changes: These can occur premenstrually, following birth, or during menopause, as a result of a lack of estrogen; they can also occur as a result of problems in thyroid function or tumors that affect the hormonal glands. These can all cause a feeling of depression. Likewise, serious, prolonged or incurable diseases often tend to bring a feeling of depression, despair, or helplessness in their wake.

Environmental causes: All environmental situations belong to this group: traumatic events such as the loss or death of a close person, separation, divorce or abandonment by a loved one, failure at work, being fired, failure in one's studies or in one's personal life, situations that induce a high level of stress, and the need to function in a stressful environment. It is interesting that depression can occur after the stress has been reduced, when the person is left without the strength and resources to carry on. In addition, loneliness also constitutes a common cause for depression. Loneliness can be objective, such as the loneliness experienced by a solitary elderly person, or subjective, in which the loneliness derives from the person's inner feeling that he cannot find friends or love, or that he does not connect with his surroundings.

A reminder of a frustrating event or loss that evokes the memory of a traumatic experience or loss that occurred in the past – when a seemingly minor event brings to mind and evokes a difficult memory from the past that was not properly processed, and brings depression in its wake.

Depression can occur in varying degrees of seriousness. There are people whose personality is diagnosed as depressive. This personality is characterized by low self-esteem, defective functioning, no enjoyment of life, problems in creating ties with people, and harsh self-criticism. These feelings accompany the person most of his life.

A cyclothymic temperament is a temperament that is characterized by sharp and rapid emotional changes that are not linked to objective reality. One day the person feels happy and full of energy and initiative, and the next, he feels depressed and lacks vigor and energy. In general, despite the sharp emotional changes, these people manage to function well in their lives.

Minor depression is a state of mild to medium depression that continues for at least two weeks, but not longer than two years. In contrast, there is a state of *major depression* (grief), which is a state of severe and profound depression that continues for at least two weeks, but not longer than two years. Its characteristics are extremely intense, so much so that the person is in a state of *anhedonia* (an inability to derive enjoyment from food, sex, being among people, and so on) and social isolation, and suffers from a sharp drop in vigor and energy, a severe lack of decisiveness, exaggerated emotions, difficulties in concentration, and fears and anxieties. Between these two states lies *dysphoria*, which is medium depression. This does not belong to the personality characteristics. It begins at a certain moment and does not continue for more than two years. This state is characterized by fears concerning the day ahead, but when the person is active – at work, with friends, having fun, etc. – he tends to feel better. When he on his own, however, the depressed feelings return.

Moreover, there is a state of *chronic depression* – major depression that continues for over two years, when the sufferer functions at an extremely low level, and waves of depressed feelings accompany him all day, with no connection to objective or environmental facts.

Among the additional states of depression that exist, there is *winter depression* – depression that occurs during the winter or at the end of the fall and disappears in the spring, and may occur at various levels of depression; *post-partum depression* – depression that occurs after birth, and is often caused by a sudden plummeting of the level of hormones in the blood. This depression generally disappears after a week or two, and can be very mild, but, having said that, a state of clinical depression, minor or major, may develop, which can continue for a long time if left untreated. Of course, there is also a state of *manic depression*, which is characterized by a highly elated mood, quick thinking, great alertness, hyperactivity, and sometimes even a feeling of arrogance and impulsive behavior, followed by a drastic switch to profound grief, depression, and an inability to function.

Essential oils have an enormous number of ways of affecting the person's state of mind. This action is explained by their effect on the limbic system in the brain, which is responsible for a very wide range of emotions. This is why the essential oils are able to exert an extremely beneficial effect on many states of depression. Having said that, it is important to remember that various cases of depression require broad and holistic treatment, including psychotherapy, orthomolecular balance (treatment with vitamins, minerals, amino acids, and other food supplements in order to regulate the body's biochemical action), and the reinforcement of the body and mind by various holistic methods, such as Bach flowers, healing, reflexology, and more. Other cases must be treated by a physician, a psychologist or a psychiatrist.

The oils that are best known for being antidepressant or uplifting are: **grapefruit, neroli, sandalwood, camphor, chamomile, clary sage** (wonderful for post-partum depression, and, in general, causes a euphoric feeling), **rose** (excellent for women, and in situations of mourning and depression as a result of loss or separation), **patchouli, petitgrain** (for light cases), **mandarine** (especially for depression resulting from a trauma – in the present or past), **vetiver** (for cases of depression that derives from a lack of estrogen), **melissa** (uplifting, helps in cases of mourning and depression as a result of loss or separation), **bergamot** (very uplifting), **marjoram** (good in states of melancholy, sorrow, and trauma, and induces a feeling of mental warmth), **jasmine** (wonderful for women), **ylang ylang** (for children), **thyme** and **rosemary** (both of which are stimulating, and contribute to promoting memory and cerebral activity, which can be adversely affected during depression).

Insomnia

Trish, a 24-year-old law student, described a very distressing situation. She wanted to sleep, but sleep simply would not come. Despite the fact that her days were very busy, and that she was genuinely tired, she could not fall asleep. She would toss and turn in bed, recall all kinds of things, go through the previous day in her head, count sheep, get out of bed, get back in again – anything but fall asleep. She felt very frustrated that her body apparently refused to obey her. Some people suggested that she take sleeping pills, but she realized that she had to get to the root of the problem, and that she could become addicted to the sleeping pills.

Insomnia and difficulties in falling asleep are very disturbing problems. In order to function in an optimal way physically, mentally, and intellectually, body and mind have to be permitted to rest. Insomnia is extremely common. About 30% of the population suffer from it. Although sleeping pills are an effective aid, they have many side effects, and can become addictive. Some people cannot actually fall asleep – a state called "difficulty in falling asleep," and others wake up very frequently or very early in the morning – a state called "ongoing insomnia."

There are many factors that can lead to insomnia and difficulty in falling asleep. Among them are nutritional factors such as stimulants: caffeine, tea, and alcohol. Birth control pills are occasionally liable to cause the problem, as are pills for treating hypertension or thyroid imbalances. In addition, there are physiological phenomena, such as stopping to breathe while sleeping, which cause the person to wake up over and over again – sometimes even without knowing it. (This induces a state of severe fatigue during the day, even though the person thinks that he had a good night's sleep; it occurs mainly with smokers and people who are overweight. It is a good idea to go to a sleep laboratory in order to have this possibility checked out.) Other factors that can lead to insomnia are a nocturnal tremor of a spastic muscle, hypoglycemia (a low blood sugar level), various pains that interfere with the person's sleep or force him to find positions that do not hurt, and so on.

Psychological factors are extremely common, and can bother a large part of the population at some time in their lives. Among these factors are depression, which can cause difficulty in falling asleep and in sleeping; early waking or sleep during the day that prevents good sleep at night; states of stress or anxiety that occurred during the day, or anxiety about the next day; excitement or emotional arousal; fear of insomnia itself or fear of sleep (because of a fear of nightmares or other psychological reasons); change of environment; or failure to adapt to the sleep environment. The latter factors generally cause difficulty in falling asleep, but later on the person manages to fall asleep. This is the same in cases of environmental disturbances, such as noise, cold or heat. Difficulty in falling asleep can also occur after a heavy meal at night or when sleeping in a poorly ventilated room. A lack of physical activity also contributes to a great extent to difficulty in falling asleep and insomnia. Of course, temporary changes in daily routine or becoming accustomed to being awake at night and sleeping in the morning may cause sleeping difficulties until they are rectified.

When treating insomnia, we must question the client and check the causes for his insomnia, which may be many and varied.

Essential oils have a marvelous ability to help in cases of insomnia. In addition to the specific oils that treat this problem – especially in the case of a client who has difficulty falling asleep or suffers from insomnia for various psychological reasons – we include oils that treat psychological problems such as anxiety, stress, depression, and so on, in the aromatic blend.

The effective ways of treating insomnia with essential oils are massage, baths, and the oil burner. The burner can be placed next to the bed at night, so long as the light of the candle does not prevent the person from falling asleep. (It is very important to check the burner's capacity beforehand to ensure that the water in it will not evaporate before the candle goes out, so as not to scorch the bottom of the saucer in the burner.) People who tend to be anxious about or aware of what is going on around them while falling asleep, and are afraid of the burning candle, must not use the oil burner prior to going to sleep, since this will only give them something else to worry about.

The aim of Trish's treatment was to help her fall asleep easily for several days consecutively in order to get her used to sleeping at the right time, so that she could wake up refreshed in the morning.

For her treatment, I chose **lavender** oil, which is an excellent oil for treating insomnia and for relaxation, **patchouli** oil, which helps calm the person down regarding worries about the next day, and **neroli** and **petitgrain** oil, which are extremely soothing, and work in tandem to treat insomnia.

The treatment was to be administered in two stages. The first was an aromatic bath before going to sleep. I asked Trish to drip three drops of **lavender** oil, two drops of **petitgrain** oil, and one drop of **neroli** oil onto a tablespoon of salt (so that the oils would mix into the bathwater better), and to add this to a tub of nice warm water. Alternatively, it is possible to use four drops of **lavender** oil and two drops of either **petitgrain** or **tangerine** oil. I asked Trish to stay in the bath for 10 to 20 minutes, while she relaxed and let herself loosen up and enjoy the pleasant bath.

After the bath, she was advised not to take a shower, but rather to dry herself lightly with a towel, and get into bed.

In bed, Trish was to ask her partner to massage her body with the massage blend. This soothing blend contained 10 cc of **almond** carrier oil, three drops of **lavender** oil, and two drops of **patchouli** oil. The massage was to be performed all over her body, using slow, gentle and soothing movements. Background music, which was relaxing or soporific, could be played in order to facilitate her falling asleep – even if this occurred during the massage. (When the massage is performed by a gentle and sensitive masseur, there is a good chance that this will happen, especially if the person is already tired after the bath.)

Trish began to use the suggested methods of treatment. The first time she tried the bath, she noticed that it made her very relaxed, and stopped her usual train of nocturnal thoughts. She simply felt too relaxed to start thinking about whether everything was ready for tomorrow, if she had done everything, and so on. After the pleasant and relaxing massage, her partner fell asleep immediately, and Trish lay sleepily in bed. Although she did not fall asleep immediately, she lay in bed almost devoid of thoughts, and after some time, her eyes closed, and she fell asleep.

The next times she repeated the treatment, she fell asleep more quickly – sometimes even during the massage. There is no doubt that the good sleep had improved her way of life to a large extent. She could now get up alert, earlier in the morning, and in a natural way, even if she had been more tired at night after a full day.

In Trish's case, in which it was necessary only to regulate her sleep patterns for a short time, aromatherapy worked very rapidly. Within a week, Trish's sleep began to settle down by itself, and she no longer needed the bath or the massage every night. Sometimes, when she thought that she would not fall asleep easily, she took a bath, or asked her partner to massage her with the essential oils. Sometimes, after only the bath, she already felt drowsy enough to fall asleep. At a certain stage, she no longer felt the need for aromatherapy.

The duration and frequency of treatment for insomnia and difficulty in falling asleep vary from person to person. Some people need the bath and the massage for a certain time or whenever they go through something that makes it difficult for them to sleep. There are others who only need part of the treatment for a very short time, or who use it only in specific cases of difficulty in falling asleep. In any event, the treatment is extremely effective and has a very good rate of success.

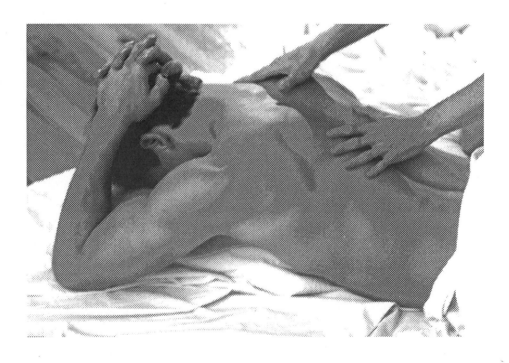

Fatigue

Rachel, a 35-year-old graphic designer and mother of three young children, had been suffering from fatigue for a long time. She would wake up early in the morning in order to get the children ready for school and kindergarten, take a shower to freshen up, and leave for her job at a newspaper. She worked for about half a day, returned home in time for the children, and then continued her workday: cooking, tidying the house, doing the laundry, and sitting with the children and helping them with their homework. Toward evening, she prepared her schedule for the next day. It was no wonder that Rachel was suffering from ongoing fatigue. She only got into bed late at night, after a heavy day's work, slept "like a log," and work up early in the morning again, for another heavy day. Since she had begun working as chief graphic designer at the newspaper – a job that placed authority, obligations, and additional tasks on her shoulders – she felt even more fatigued for most of the day. She was investing more energy in it than she had in the past, and, at the same time, trying to ensure that everything "went like clockwork" at home. Her husband came home from work late, and, while he tried to help her with the housework and the kids, Rachel still carried most of the burden.

There was no doubt that Rachel's attempt at being "Superwoman" both at home and at work was leaving its mark on her. The more the fatigue accumulated, the more indifferent and insensible Rachel felt during the day. She did not have patience; she tried to do everything quickly, sometimes automatically, and this just created more work for her. Sometimes she had headaches in the early afternoon, after making lunch for the kids, and during those hours she experienced a noticeable drop in energy. The fatigue she suffered from also left its mark on her work process, since she sometimes felt unfocused, and things that usually took only a short time to do took longer and stretched out like elastic because of her fatigue and lack of concentration.

Fatigue, as opposed to exhaustion or debility, which are more serious conditions that have to be examined and treated immediately, is a very common problem. In most cases, it stems from concerted physical or mental activity over a long time, hard work, a lack of proper sleep, or – very common – from states of stress and mental tension. Moreover, fatigue can stem from physiological causes such as thyroid problems, incorrect nutrition that does not supply the body with the necessary vitamins and minerals, problems of sleep and falling asleep, hypoglycemia (a low blood sugar level), or sleep disturbances that the person is not aware of, such as stopping to breathe while sleeping, which causes him to wake up over and over again, or the nocturnal tremor of a spastic muscle. When it is suspected that the fatigue stems from one of these causes, it must be examined thoroughly in a sleep laboratory or through medical tests that measure sugar level or thyroid function. Of course, fatigue may also be a result of various diseases that exhaust the person, or as the after-effects of a disease (for instance, after flu), and then every case must be dealt with individually in order to relieve the pains or the disease.

Many stimulating and invigorating essential oils are used in aromatherapy. However, for treating fatigue, we mainly use soothing oils and an effective remedy – rest. When fatigue derives from mental stress, or, as in Rachel's case, from the need to do everything perfectly, in keeping with a true perfectionist, ignoring her body's needs, we are likely to achieve the opposite results if we stimulate the body to action.

The use of stimulating oils in conjunction with the techniques of stimulation through massage or reflexology is recommended for the treatment of mild fatigue, especially when it is not ongoing, and for some reason the person has to wake up and function normally but has no time to rest. However, when it is a case of ongoing fatigue, our aim is to calm the body down and demand that the person give his body the rest it needs in order not to reach a state of utter exhaustion.

Although Rachel had difficulty accepting the fact that she was wearing herself out, I explained that she had to give herself hours of rest, preferably during the afternoon, when she felt the drop in energy, as well as good, undisturbed, and satisfying sleep at night.

I suggested a very effective, refreshing, and fortifying treatment with aromatherapy. During the afternoon, when she felt her strength waning, she was advised to take an aromatic bath. Alternatively, if she preferred, she could take the bath before going to sleep at night.

She was to drip three drops of **lavender** oil, two drops of **pine** oil, two drops of **neroli** oil, and one drop of **melissa** oil onto one and a half or two tablespoons of salt, and mix it into the bathwater.

I asked Rachel to lie in the bath for 15 to 20 minutes, allowing herself to relax and empty her mind of everyday worries. She could take an aromatic bath every day, several times a week, or as she felt was necessary.

Another stage in the treatment was the aromatic massage. This massage was to be performed all over the body, but a massage of the back and chest area would also suffice. She was to be massaged with essential oils by a qualified masseur three times during the first week of treatment (in such a case, it is advisable to have the bath and the massage on alternate days) and once a week from the second week onward for a certain period of time. She could have a partial body massage of the back and chest daily (except on days when she had a full massage).

Rachel wanted to have a massage in the clinic twice during the first week, instead of three times, because she could not find the time to come for the massage three times. (Remember that it is not always necessary to undergo treatment in a clinic for fatigue. The massage can be performed by a partner or friend at home.) I asked her to ask her husband to perform the body massage – full or partial – on the days she did not get a massage.

I prepared a massage blend that contained 30 cc of **almond** carrier oil, five drops of **lavender** oil, five drops of **neroli** oil, and five drops of **pine** oil.

Note that **neroli** oil, which is used in both the massage and the bath blends, is phototoxic, and after applying it, the person must not expose himself to the sun for 12 hours from the time of application. In cases in which exposure to the sun cannot be avoided, for various reasons, it is advisable to substitute **marjoram** or **clary sage** oil for the **neroli**.

In addition to the baths and massages, I suggested that Rachel use an oil burner containing 12 drops of one or more of the following essential oils: **ylang ylang**, **lavender**, **pine**, **neroli**, **marjoram**, **bergamot**, and **rose**. In the blend I prepared for Rachel's oil burner, I used the following pure oils (that is, without a carrier oil): **lavender**, **pine**, **neroli**, and **marjoram**.

I advised Rachel to use the burner several times a day, preferably during the hours she did not work, and during the time she allotted to herself for resting, in order to facilitate the rest. This is very important, considering that although Rachel was so tired, she had a hard time really and truly resting and relaxing, since she found it difficult to put her everyday tasks aside. Even during the hours she sat down to rest, thoughts of the obligations and tasks she had to complete during the day raced through her head, and she was unable to rest fully.

The massages she was given gave her a fortifying, relaxing, and encouraging feeling. She decided to have the baths in the afternoon, and permitted herself to pay a young girl to look after the children and help them with their homework while she relaxed peacefully in the bathtub and then went into her bedroom to rest for two hours. During the day, she used the oil burner, and before going to sleep, on the days she did not have a massage, she asked her husband to massage her with the blend of oils. Sometimes her husband performed a full massage. When he was also tired, Rachel made do with a partial massage of her back, neck, and chest.

She did not have to wait long for the results. Shortly after beginning the treatment, Rachel began to feel more fortified and refreshed. Not much later, she learned how to permit herself to rest and relax. The baths, the massages, and the use of the oil burner significantly reduced the level of stress she was subjected to during the day. Her headaches and concentration problems began to disappear. She noticed that as a result of the use of the oils, she was sleeping better and more fully, she could really rest with an empty mind, and this rest recharged her energy supplies. Afterwards she was able to continue the day better and was more refreshed.

Since she was vital and energetic during the day, she did the things she had to do more efficiently and quickly. (Before, she had experienced a drop in energy that caused a lack in concentration, and she worked slowly and rather indifferently). Now she could concentrate her energy better and more correctly and get through more work in a shorter time, which, of course, meant that she had more time for herself.

In an effective and meaningful way, aromatherapy helped Rachel to extricate herself from the vicious circle of fatigue and self-exhaustion, to learn how to listen to her body properly, and to act in accordance with its needs. Today, although she no longer suffers from fatigue, she still takes relaxing baths with essential oils to calm down, feel good, and raise her energy level.

The sexual and reproductive system

For hundreds of years, essential oils have played a central role in the treatment of the sexual system because of their marvelous properties in this field. Many ointments that were made from essential oils hundreds of years ago exploited these properties, especially the aphrodisiac property (for attracting and arousing the opposite sex) which is found in several essential oils. Since human sexuality is linked directly to state of mind, the essential oils, with their welcome action both on the psychological and the physical levels, reveal themselves to be wonderfully effective in the treatment of sexual problems.

The range of problems in the sexual and reproductive system that essential oils can help with is extremely broad: from menstrual problems, including cramps and irregular periods, and so on, to treating sexual problems whose source is psychological – such as a lack of confidence in one's sexuality, tension and anxiety, hormonal problems, and menopausal problems, to the reinforcement of the sexual system and sexual arousal. It is clear that in the sexual realm, the treatment of the symptoms of the problems (for instance, impotence, frigidity, premature ejaculation, and so on, that sometimes stem from other problems) is just as important as treating the problem and its cause.

The aphrodisiac (sexual stimulant) property that is attributed to several of the essential oils is not merely a rumor or wishful thinking. On the contrary: sometimes, their action in this realm is so powerful that it is surprising in its intensity. As a rule, every intimate encounter that is accompanied by an oil burner emitting the fragrances of aphrodisiac oils, let alone an aromatic bath or a mutual body massage with essential oils, is far more fascinating and enjoyable than one without it.

The action of the oils is also relevant to the hormonal and the nervous systems, and while it strengthens the body and the tone of the sexual system, it makes the oils into a tool that helps and supports many problems.

Various problems, such as menopausal symptoms, male impotence, frigidity, prostate problems, and so on, require comprehensive treatment, and often medical intervention or psychotherapy. However, the addition of aromatherapy can strengthen and support the comprehensive treatment.

It would take too long to describe the range of problems and symptoms in the sexual and reproductive system and the clients treated by essential oils, so I will describe in detail only the central ones – treatment of menstrual cramps and premenstrual syndrome (PMS), menopausal problems, and increasing passion and sexual arousal. Many other problems and symptoms have been discussed in other chapters of this book – for instance, the fact that stress has a negative effect on sexual energy, and that the reduction of stress improves sexual function; hypertension can lead to problems of erection, and treatment can solve this problem, and so on.

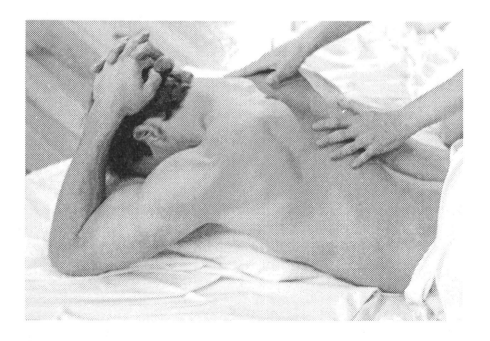

Premenstrual tension (PMS)

Let's begin with a few remarks about the monthly period in general:

There are many problems that the use of essential oils can help solve.

For irregular periods, bath and massage blends can be used. The following oils are suitable for treating this problem: **chamomile**, **rose**, and **fennel**. **Melissa**, too, helps normalize the periods.

For balancing the amount of bleeding, **juniper** oil, which is also effective for treating conditions in which there is too little menstrual bleeding, can be used. **Peppermint** oil can also be used for this purpose.

For treating heavy menstrual bleeding, one or more of the following essential oils should be included: **yarrow**, **peppermint**, **sage**, **chamomile**, **camphor**, **cypress**, **rose**, and **clary sage**.

In order to induce a period that is late, we use **juniper** and **lavender** in the blend.

For treating a painful and congested period, **fennel**, **cypress**, and **geranium** oils are recommended.

If there is an accumulation of premenstrual fluids, **geranium** and **fennel** oil can be included in the blend.

Amenorrhea (absence of a period) requires in-depth and comprehensive treatment, since this problem is sometimes a warning sign of serious conditions of a hormonal, physical, or mental imbalance. (Anorexia, for instance, is characterized by amenorrhea.) Aromatherapy can be very effective when combined with holistic treatment, psychotherapy, and medical treatment, as required. The essential oils that are recommended are **cinnamon**, **juniper**, and **clary sage**.

As a rule, the essential oils that are considered to balance hormonal action are **geranium**, **fennel**, **clary sage**, and **yarrow**, but in such a case, it is extremely important to get to the root of the problem and not just treat the symptoms.

Laura, a 23-year-old woman, came for treatment as a result of her husband's entreaties. A tall, thin, very good-looking woman, well groomed and a bit bashful entered the clinic rather hesitantly. After introducing herself, she told me that she worked at home, typing papers for students, had got married two years previously, and that her marriage was happy and fulfilling. She hastened to add:

"I don't really think you can help me. I simply take a pill, lie in bed for a while, and wait for it to pass."

"Wait for what to pass?" I asked, because she still hadn't told me what her problem was.

In a few minutes, Laura presented a long and painful sketch of the menstrual cramps and PMS symptoms that had plagued her since the very first time she got her period – at age thirteen and a half. The cramps seized hold of her and would not let go. After her period arrived, the pains would concentrate in the area of her lower abdomen and lower back, sometimes accompanied by headaches and pressure in her temples. In addition, she was bothered by her change of mood during her period and especially several days beforehand. (This was the main thing that bothered her husband and made him beg her to come for treatment.)

According to Laura, she was generally a calm and quiet type of person who did not tend to be easily offended or raise her voice. I was struck by her obvious gentleness and her quiet, calm tone, as well as by her body language, which, except for a bit of shyness and lack of confidence due to a meeting with an unfamiliar professional, radiated tranquillity and refinement. However, as she herself described, before her period and sometimes a few days after getting it, she tended to be irritable, was easily offended, got upset about everything, and reacted angrily and impatiently to her husband's smallest request. Her moods chopped and changed, zigzagging sometimes between a disturbing feeling of depression to inner agitation. In addition, the cramps she got at the beginning of her period caused her a great deal of anguish.

Generally speaking, Laura would take pills to relieve her period pains (one to three), but they only took effect three-quarters of an hour after being taken, and they did not relieve the pains entirely. She preferred to lie down and rest – and this interfered with her normal functioning. She wanted treatment that would help dispel her irritation and hypersensitivity.

Besides period pains, Laura's health was good; she had not undergone any surgery, or had any fractures, etc., and her general mood was good. After a slightly more in-depth interview, she admitted that she sometimes suffered from mild insomnia, which worsened a few days before her period – but not too much – and she did not take any medications for it – just "waited for sleep to come."

Period pains, often accompanied by changes in the emotional state, are caused by uterine contractions during menstruation and by hormonal changes. Period pains usually occur once the period has arrived.

One to two weeks before the period, irritation, depression, intolerance, and other emotional phenomena may occur, and this complex is known as premenstrual syndrome (PMS). About one-third of all women suffer from PMS or from menstrual cramps. The symptoms are many and varied, and include a large range of phenomena such as anxiety, impatience, mood swings, tension, irritation, depression, weepiness, forgetfulness, a feeling of confusion, insomnia, increased appetite (sometimes in the form of a craving for either "sweet" or "salty"), headaches, fatigue, dizziness, and in extreme cases fainting, palpitations, fluid retention, weight gain, breast sensitivity, swollen limbs, and a swollen abdomen.

The phenomena of PMS and period pains, like other problems related to the monthly period – congestion, heavy bleeding, irregularity, and so on – can be treated with essential oils. The success of the treatment with the oils is individual and depends on the seriousness of the problem and its causes. In certain cases, the treatment with essential oils is more effective when it is combined with holistic or medical treatment.

There are many oils that treat a broad range of menstrual problems. A large portion of the oils that treat problems of period pains also treat additional facets of the sexual and reproductive system.

Yarrow oil is very suitable for a general treatment of menstrual problems, for period pains, and for menopause, and most of its efficient action stems from the fact that it balances hormonal action.

Geranium oil, which is also thought to balance hormonal action, can also help in cases of premenstrual fluid retention, as well as in PMS and congestion during periods and menopause.

Melissa oil, which has significant effects on the psychological aspect, helps normalize unbalanced periods, relieves period pains, and is suitable for treatment of irregular ovulation.

Clary sage oil is effective in treating period pains and premenstrual tension, as well as heavy bleeding, and it helps balance the action of the female hormonal system.

Jasmine oil is one of the most famous oils for treating the sexual system. It reinforces the system, helps PMS, and meets almost all the needs and aspects of the sexual system. Furthermore, it strengthens, balances, and tones the system, in addition to being a very effective aphrodisiac.

Marjoram oil is very helpful in treating premenstrual pains, as well as states of sexual imbalance (powerful sexual drive, nymphomania, and excessive masturbation).

Fennel oil, which stimulates estrogen production, is good for PMS, menopause, regulating periods, making the skin strong and elastic, and strengthening and balancing the hormonal system.

Chamomile oil, which is anti-inflammatory, is good for all inflammatory states. Moreover, it is effective in treating PMS, stress and depression resulting from hormonal imbalance, and menopause. Its properties of relaxing and "mental work" are very important in treating these type of problems.

We use **cypress** and **rosewood** oils for treating period pains and PMS.

As I said before, treatment with essential oils is a holistic treatment that attempts to treat – to the best of its ability – all the symptoms that are bothering the client, the mild ones as well as the serious ones, in addition to focusing on the main problem.

When I treated Laura, I decided to focus on the three following symptoms:
1. Her period pains, which included pains in her back and lower abdomen, headaches, and a general uncomfortable feeling.
2. The psychological symptoms that occurred as a result of the hormonal changes during her period – hypersensitivity, agitation, a feeling of general discomfort and intolerance.
3. I also had to relate to her problem of insomnia, which should not be taken lightly, even if it only occurred infrequently.

For the holistic and inclusive treatment I chose the following essential oils: **chamomile**, **cypress**, and **neroli**.

Chamomile oil is antispasmodic, that is, it soothes cramps, and thus helps soothe the uterine cramps that cause period pains. Moreover, it is an analgesic, and helps relieve a broad range of mental states, such as depression, hypersensitivity, anxiety and tension, and on the physical level it is known to help in cases of headaches, muscle pains, and, of course, period pains. For this reason, this oil would help Laura both on the physical and on the mental plane. **Neroli** oil is known for its soothing properties, for being antispasmodic, for helping in cases of muscle pains, and for possessing a broad range of properties on the mental level – it alleviates anxiety and depression, is very soothing and invokes tranquillity, and moreover helps in cases of insomnia. **Cypress** oil was added to balance the blend and because of its efficiency in alleviating pains and period pains.

The effective ways of dealing with the pains, in addition to aromatherapy, are by physical activity, which can relieve premenstrual symptoms, and by warming the painful areas with a hot-water bottle. Aromatherapy treatment includes warm baths and massage. The oil burner is used mainly for treating the psychological aspects of PMS.

For the first stage of Laura's treatment, I suggested that she use a blend of oils in the bath. To this end, I prepared a blend of pure oils (without carrier oils), consisting of **chamomile**, **cypress**, and **neroli** oils. Laura was to drip 5-7 drops of the blend into the bathwater, and lie in the water for 15-20 minutes. I recommended that she have the bath before going to sleep, since it contained phototoxic **neroli** oil, which meant that she cannot expose her skin to the sun for 12 hours after use. She could get into the bath according to how she felt – when she felt strong pains or emotional phenomena – but then too she was to ensure not to expose herself to sunshine afterwards. (Of course, the bath was meant for the days before and after the period itself, according to how Laura felt.)

The second stage of the treatment was a massage with essential oils. This is of great importance in relieving period pains. Through massage, it is possible to warm the painful areas (the abdomen and the lower back, in Laura's case), thereby soothing the cramps and the pains. Moreover, the massage blend would contribute to calming Laura down, and it was a good idea to use it on the days preceding her period, too, even if there were no pains then, in order to soothe the emotional symptoms.

I prepared the massage blend from 30 cc of **almond** carrier oil (cold-pressed **sunflower** oil can be used equally well), six drops of **chamomile** oil, and nine drops of **cypress** oil. Laura could perform the massage herself by massaging the area of the lower abdomen, and her husband could help her massage her lower back. Since it was a matter of a local massage only, she could massage the area every time she felt the need. This amount was sufficient for many local massages. (For preparing a smaller amount, a third of the amount of carrier oil and the indicated essential oils can be used.)

As a blend for the oil burner, whose aim was to help balance Laura's emotional state during her period and especially beforehand, I could use altogether 12 drops of the following oils: **geranium**, **jasmine**, **marjoram**, **melissa**, **cypress**, **clary sage**, **chamomile**, **lavender**, **neroli**, and **fennel**. I suggested that Laura use **chamomile**, **neroli**, **cypress**, and **lavender** (since the first three were in the blend for her bath and massage, and **lavender** oil is very effective for treating insomnia and also for the headaches she suffered from occasionally – it could be exchanged for **melissa** oil, which also helps relieve headaches).

Laura began to take the baths about a week before getting her period, the moment she felt that she was getting out of emotional balance. To her joy, a few days later – after taking a soothing bath every evening – she discovered that she felt a significant improvement in her mood. At the same time, she used the oil burner, sometimes even two or three times a day, when she felt in a particularly bad mood, and as a result felt a great deal of relief. She was less sensitive, less easy to irritate and offend, less agitated, more tolerant, and reacted more easily to emotional changes, instead of reacting in an extreme manner as she had in the past. After her period arrived, and the exhausting pains began, she continued using the oil burner and doing the massages (once or twice a day she massaged her lower abdomen) and these soothed her pains and lower abdominal cramps significantly. She felt that the massage warmed the painful area, soothed it, and relieved it. In the evening, she asked her husband to massage her lower back for a few minutes, which would help her sleep better and without pain. Her headaches, too, were relieved mainly as a result of the use of the oil burner, and since she used the oils before going to sleep, and because of the general feeling of relaxation afforded by the daily use of the oil burner, her sleep was much better, and she fell asleep easily and woke up refreshed in the morning.

Laura was grateful for the solution provided by the essential oils. For the first time in her life, she felt that she could get through those two awful weeks of unbalanced emotional symptoms and irksome pains much more easily. After a few months of using the essential oil in the days preceding and during her period, the symptoms themselves began to be less intense and disturbing, and her need to use aromatherapy decreased in frequency – in addition to a decrease in pain and emotional changes.

Menopause

Brenda, a 49-year-old self-employed graphic designer, mother of three grown children, came for treatment with aromatherapy because of a disturbing problem that is extremely common among women of that age group. Brenda was at the beginning of menopause, and she was suffering from many disturbing symptoms that go hand in hand with that stage of life. Since her period had not yet stopped completely, she was suffering from irregular and unbalanced periods, as well as from period pains. In addition, she was plagued by hot flashes that had begun to occur from time to time, generally accompanied by sweating and flushing, and this made her uncomfortable and embarrassed when she was in company.

Brenda was especially bothered by mood swings. She told me that she was a person who could cope with difficulties and physical pain with relative ease, and so long as her mood was good and she was optimistic and full of life, even the physical symptoms of menopause could not bring her down. However, when the mood swings began to occur the previous year, together with irregular periods, she had a hard time coping. By nature, she had always been a very energetic and lively person, and now she occasionally felt a lack of energy for no apparent reason. Sometimes she even felt exhausted as a result of a drop in energy, which bothered her at work, distracted her, and interfered with her concentration. She would get through those times by lying down for an hour or two, until she felt a bit better and her strength returned to her. She occasionally felt a slight depression, which bothered her a lot, since she had never experienced feelings of depression before. In addition, her general sensitivity increased greatly, and she found herself offended, upset, or crying for no particular reason.

From the psychological point of view, she was disturbed by the changes that were taking place in her body, and the intensity with which she had begun to feel unwell (mainly because she had previously been a healthy person). In addition to all those symptoms, her libido, which had been normal and constant, had begun to decease, which contributed to the vicious circle and to her feeling that she was becoming "less feminine and less sexy." The gradual decrease in her sexual desire was causing conflicts between her and her husband, who thought that she no longer desired him. Although he understood the processes that she was going through, it was difficult for him to internalize the situation and adapt to it, and it was also clear that Brenda herself felt disturbed by the fact that her libido had decreased.

Although she considered menopause to be natural and inevitable, deep inside her she felt vulnerable and unsure of her femininity, even though she could explain this feeling. She was trying to maintain her health by eating correctly and engaging in physical activity (which is also important for preventing osteoporosis, a bone-thinning disease that all post-menopausal women are prone to; it is important to begin to strengthen the bones and improve their density through regular physical exercise from age 35!). Besides the menopausal symptoms, Brenda did not suffer from health problems, but she mentioned that in the past three months, she had been having difficulty falling asleep and sleeping, even after a long, tiring day of work.

The term "menopause" refers to the time between the end of a woman's fertility and a total absence of menstruation. The duration of menopause can be for a few months to a few years. On average, age 48 is considered to be the beginning age for menopause, but that, of course, is only a statistical average, and there are women who begin menopause at 40, and others who begin after 50.

This transition period presents women with several new problems, since both the regular monthly sex hormone and ovum production is disrupted. As a result, the monthly cycle is disrupted, and becomes irregular until it ceases completely. At the same time, the state of hormonal imbalance causes certain physical and emotional problems.

It must be remembered that menopause is completely natural, and it is part of women's normal development. However, in Western culture, several negative connotations have been attached to it, and it has been referred to as "the period of aging," a name that angers many women. In other more traditional cultures – often called "primitive" according to the condescending Western definition – this period is in fact believed to be a "gift" to the woman, who terminates her period of fertility and with it the never-ending need to look after children, and gradually assumes the status of "an elder of the tribe," whose wisdom and experience are revered. In extreme religious societies that also approve the birth of large numbers of children, there are women who see menopause as a time of well-being, which symbolizes the beginning of a new era in which the woman can devote more time to herself and less to taking care of offspring.

It is important to mention that the way in which a woman perceives this stage – whether she sees it as something natural, sometimes even useful, or if she sees it as a sign of "old age" or diminished femininity – is extremely significant. The more naturally a woman accepts this stage, the greater her chances that the symptoms and syndromes that accompany it will be less disturbing.

We cannot ignore the symptoms that accompany menopause, however intense they may or may not be. About 75% of the women who go through this transition period experience mental and physical changes. Some feel these changes and symptoms to a large degree, sometimes to the point of disrupting their everyday life. Among the common symptoms are sudden hot flashes, sudden flushing as a result of the hot flash, sweating, palpitations, changes in libido – sometimes dryness and soreness in the vagina that make sexual intercourse difficult – joint pains and headaches, as well as a broad range of emotional imbalance, such as a feeling of depression, agitation, anxiety, a lack of concentration, a lack of energy, and sleep problems. These symptoms can last from a few weeks to several years.

In general, women go through this stage naturally, despite the difficulties, but in cases in which the symptoms are particularly disturbing, a woman is treated with hormone replacement therapy (HRT) in the form of pills that resemble contraceptive pills, or skin patches (or by means of a vaginal ointment) that contain a combination of the hormones progesterone and estrogen, or each hormone separately. The treatment helps to eliminate the symptoms. Many women (as well as many doctors) are not in a great hurry to avail themselves of hormonal treatment, since it is relatively new and there is not sufficient information about its long-term side effects.

In many cases of menopausal problems, holistic treatment – such as reflexology, Bach flower remedies, Shiatsu, herbal remedies, aromatherapy, and so on – can be extremely beneficial.

In aromatherapy, there are many oils that are used for moderating and easing menopausal symptoms, and constitute a significant mental support for the broad range of emotional and psychological phenomena that accompany this process. Moreover, the essential oils also help stimulate the libido, which is likely to decrease somewhat during this period, and help with the sleep problems, hypersensitivity, mood swings and depression that may accompany menopause.

Among the oils that are used for treating menopausal symptoms, the following are known to be very effective:

Vetiver oil is one of the best-known oils for treating menopausal problems. **Vetiver** oil works like estrogen, so it is good for a broad range of menopausal symptoms, the shortage of estrogen and depression of menopause, which in many cases stem from a drop or changes in the body's estrogen level. **Vetiver** oil also calms and relieves states of anger and irritation and helps release tensions (it is wonderful in the bath), and stimulates cell and tissue regeneration.

Fennel oil, too, which is known to balance hormone activity generally, is effective in treating the shortage of estrogen, since it stimulates estrogen production, helps a bit in regulating irregular monthly periods, reinforces and balances the hormonal system, adds elasticity and strength to the skin, and is suitable for mature skin – which makes it very effective in treating the cosmetic aspects of this stage.

For treating the emotional aspects of menopause, **chamomile** oil does excellent work. It is effective in treating mood swings and depression resulting from a menopausal hormonal imbalance, soothes agitation and moderates hypersensitivity.

Yarrow oil, which balances hormonal activity, is very effective in treating a broad range of menopausal symptoms that stem from the hormonal changes wrought by this stage, and it is also effective in treating conditions of weakness that occur during menopause.

Geranium oil also balances hormonal activity, relieves pains and sensitivities during menopause, and it is wonderful for use in massages and baths because of its cosmetic properties, and its contribution to freshening and strengthening the skin (this oil is also superb for treating mature skin). It is good for attaining emotional balance.

Sage oil, which has an estrogenic character, is also suitable for all menopausal problems, but, as we said before, its level of toxicity is high, so only experienced professional aromatherapists should administer treatment with it.

Clary sage, a relative of the previous oil, also helps balance the hormonal system, and, in addition, treats other menopausal problems such as mental exhaustion, a feeling of weakness, depression and tension. It also helps strengthen the uterus.

Other oils that can be suitable for treating menopausal effects are **rose** and **jasmine**. These oils, that are considered to be supporting oils, reinforce and benefit the sexual system (both female and male). Many women testify that these oils help them feel more feminine and sexy. Indeed, both of these oils are renowned aphrodisiacs, and they help balance the emotional state in a way that permits sexual arousal, which may be "dormant" for emotional reasons. **Rose** oil is known as "the queen of the feminine oils," and it helps treat conditions of a lack of confidence in one's femininity and in one's feminine sexuality. This oil and **jasmine** oil, too, balance and reinforce the sexual system. **Rose** oil is also thought to be a tonic for the uterus, and it is important to include it in treatments for the prevention of a prolapsed uterus. These oils are also wonderful for treating, freshening, reviving, and reinforcing the skin.

Melissa oil, too, with its broad range of actions in the mental realm, can be suitable for a blend for treating menopausal problems. **Melissa** oil is also effective in helping to improve concentration, which may decline a bit during this period. Moreover, it fortifies sexual prowess, and also improves the skin and serves as a regenerator (encourages the growth of new cells).

The treatment I prepared for Brenda included massage (twice a week for the first week, and afterwards once a week), baths, and an oil burner. For the massage blend, I used 20 cc of **almond** carrier oil, 5 cc of **apricot kernel** carrier oil, and 5 cc of **wheatgerm** carrier oil. The essential oils I chose for Brenda's treatment were **rose** (three drops), **chamomile** (four drops), **vetiver** (three drops), and **yarrow** (four drops). (**Yarrow** and **vetiver** oils have odors that are not universally liked. It is important to check first whether the client finds the fragrances pleasant and to balance the blend carefully, since in this case, the blend contains many oils with dominant or powerful odors.)

For the bath blend, I used the same oils without the carrier oils, and this blend was also used for the oil burner.

I suggested that Brenda take a bath three times a week, and light the oil burner several times a day, especially when she felt a drop or a change in her mood. For a more effective treatment of hot flashes, I referred Brenda for treatment with herbal remedies – which has frequently had very good results.

During the first week, Brenda felt relief, especially in the mental realm. She still experienced energy depletion, but in a milder form, and she felt some relief in her hypersensitivity, and a little more vitality during the day. She went to a herbal remedy practitioner for treatment of her hot flashes, but she had not yet felt any results.

Gradually, as the treatment went on, Brenda's frequent mood swings and feelings of weakness, agitation, and hypersensitivity became less and less frequent. She felt calmer and more tranquil, and, by lighting the oil burner before going to sleep, she improved her sleep substantially. Gradually, her hot flashes became milder and shorter, and the redness that spread over her face during the hot flashes almost disappeared. To her joy, the hot flashes became far less annoying than they had been previously. Her level of vitality also improved amazingly, and the feelings of depression she had experienced became less frequent, milder, and passed quickly. Brenda's sex drive, which had waned largely because of her menopausal symptoms and her emotional state, began to be aroused and become balanced.

Her period, which was in its final stages, did not become regular, but when it came, there were no pains, it was much milder and more balanced, and Brenda went through it very easily.

By persisting with the treatment, Brenda felt much calmer, more tranquil and serene during the entire day, and she began to devote more time to herself, to her personal grooming, and to other things that interested her. When her husband offered to massage her with essential oils in the evening, before going to sleep, she discovered that her libido, which had been non-existent for some time, was becoming aroused, and she felt greater passion than ever. Since this experimental massage had been a huge success, the couple began to spend a lot of time massaging each other with essential oils (I prepared a blend that was tailor-made for her husband, at Brenda's request), and there was an appreciable improvement in their sex life.

Brenda began to perceive the stage she was going through as a springboard to doing the things she had always wanted to do but had never been able to do in the past because of a lack of time and energy. However, now her children had left home and she could permit herself to work less intensely, which left her a lot more free time for herself.

Now that she felt that the disturbing emotional changes were hardly bothering her, and from the physical point of view she felt full of life and energy, she began to devote time to things that had interested her in the past – painting and sculpture – and she registered for some courses. She also began to devote more time to her relationship with her husband.

Brenda continued using the essential oils even after we had finished the 25 massage treatments at the clinic, since she felt that they had contributed enormously to the improvement in her mood, health and feeling. Thanks to her awareness, menopause, which is considered difficult and distressing by so many women, became enjoyable, fortifying and full of potential.

Sexual arousal

Lori, a 27-year-old divorcée, a music teacher by profession, came for treatment with aromatherapy as a result of a drop in her libido and problems during intercourse. During her marriage, she had enjoyed sex with her husband, and was easily satisfied. The problem began about five months after her divorce.

Lori met a man she liked a lot, and felt that they were compatible. Her new partner was also divorced, without children, and wanted to start a new chapter in his life. He fell in love with Lori at first sight. Lori thought that she desired him and wanted to have intimate relations with him, but once they were in bed, she felt her libido "dwindling," and soon her passion had waned, and she was no longer interested in sex. Deep inside her, Lori felt nervous and anxious about having sex (more subconsciously than consciously).

Lori understood that something was "not quite right" here, since she had never had a problem with libido and sexual arousal before. For her, it was another sign – one of many – that she was still in a state of crisis following her divorce. After this insight, Lori began psychotherapy. After a few meetings with the psychotherapist, Lori understood, among other things, some of the feelings that prevented her from feeling passion or desire for intercourse, or caused her passion to wane. It was a group of factors that included guilt feelings (toward her ex-husband), a feeling that she was doing something "wrong," anxiety and nervousness about the sexual act itself, and other feelings. Through psychotherapy, she could overcome the divorce crisis as well as other problems. In the meanwhile, however, until the lengthy treatment process came to an end or showed "results," Lori wanted effective help for her problem of a lack of libido.

Problems of a lack of libido or a general lack of sexual arousal before and during intercourse are complex phenomena that can be brought on by a broad range of causes, some physiological and some psychological (the latter are sometimes more significant). The situation is not always critical, for instance, with couples who feel "bored" and experience a drop in libido after having had sex with each other for a very long time. Sometimes, the situation stems simply from daily worries: nervousness or difficulty in relaxing and forgetting everything and simply concentrating on the pleasurable sensation. When the problems are physical (such as vaginismus, a burning sensation in the vagina, pains during intercourse that cause a fear of sex, etc.) or psychological (and these are numerous and range from sexual traumas or a feeling of guilt during sex to a fear of losing control, etc.), aromatherapy must be used in conjunction with the appropriate holistic, medical or psychological treatment.

The contribution of the essential oils to increasing libido is exceptionally successful. Besides the calmness that they induce – and this in itself treats a whole category of problems that mar enjoyable sex, such as tension, pressure, anxiety, an inability to relax and let go, and so on – the essential oils have amazing properties regarding sexual arousal.

These oils are called *aphrodisiac oils*, and they have been used for hundreds of years. Over time, these oils have been linked to many tales about their ability to attract the opposite sex and to arouse sexual desire. Although these are tales, whoever uses these oils is likely to discover that there is a great deal of truth in them.

Among the known aphrodisiac oils, some can affect one particular person more, while others have a powerful effect on another person. There are many essential oils with a sexually arousing action, and the most famous among them are **rose**, **jasmine**, **ylang ylang**, **cypress**, **vetiver**, **ginger**, **clary sage**, **neroli**, **celery**, **sandalwood**, **patchouli**, **parsley**, **black pepper**, **clove**, **thyme**, **cardamon**, and **basil**.

In order to arouse sexual passion and desire, we can use the essential oils in any number of ways, as far as our imagination allows us. A massage or an aromatic bath, one or both, are the most common. An oil burner that fills the room with pleasant and arousing fragrances can also greatly enhance pleasure and desire.

However, we have to remember not to use undiluted oils in a massage, and it is important to know that condoms must not come into contact with the essential oils, since the latter damage the rubber.

I suggested to Lori that she use essential oils in three ways: in an oil burner, in the bath, and in massages. To this end, I prepared her a really "explosive" blend of the following aphrodisiac oils: **absolute rose** (very expensive, and wonderfully effective), which, besides its significant contribution to increasing the libido, also reinforces confidence in femininity and sexuality (not for nothing is this oil called "queen of the oils"!), and in Lori's case, effective in helping her overcome the feeling of crisis and separation that she was experiencing as a result of her divorce. **Jasmine** oil is also a very luxurious oil, and is thought to be a wonderful sexual stimulant. It is a soothing oil, and helps reduce pressure and anxiety, which is very important in treatment for increasing sexual desire. The third oil I chose was the fragrant **patchouli** oil, which is also a wonderful sexual stimulant, as well as being very soothing. It helps relax tensions and release anxiety.

For the massage blend, I used 30 cc of **almond** carrier oil, to which I added four drops of **patchouli** oil, two drops of **rose** oil, and three drops of **absolute jasmine** oil. (**Absolute rose** and **absolute jasmine**, that is, the pure and expensive oils, may be very concentrated and powerful in their odor, so only a small amount need be used in a blend, according to the fragrance.) I prepared a similar blend, without the carrier oil, for use in the bath and the oil burner.

The first time Lori decided to use the blend I had prepared for her, she was a bit nervous. She rested a while before getting into a warm bath – alone – into which she had dripped a few drops of the blend. She lay in the tub for 20 minutes, after which she felt fantastic – physically and mentally.

Her partner, who was well aware of her problem and stood by her all the way, was more than ready to start massaging Lori's body with the massage blend. They agreed that if the bath, the gentle and arousing massage that he was going to give her, and the warming fragrances that filled the room "did not do their work," Lori would enjoy a nice massage that would not develop into full intercourse. On the other hand, if the oils did indeed live up to their reputation, endless possibilities lay before them.

Lori's partner began to massage her body gently. It didn't take long for the massage to become an erotic massage, and I leave the rest to your imagination. In short, Lori was surprised at how the oils helped her open up sexually.

There is no doubt that the psychological treatment Lori underwent, as well as her partner's support, contributed in a large part to the success of the treatment. Lori reported that since that day, she has not stopped using the essential oils, and has found additional and novel ways to enjoy their marvelous action.

Now, long after she and her partner began their relationship, and most of her emotional problems have been solved, including her drop in libido, Lori's partner has also begun to enjoy the wonderful properties of the oils, and they try different blends and new aphrodisiac oils in order to increase their fun, pleasure and sexual satisfaction.

Treating the elderly and frail-care patients with essential oils

Treatment with essential oils is really a heaven-sent blessing for the elderly and for frail-care patients who suffer from serious diseases and spend most of their time in bed. Frail-care treatment generally focuses on facilitating everyday functions and on the physical treatment of problems, and sometimes ignores the psychological aspects, not to mention the warmth, support, and mental help that the elderly and frail-care patients need. These people go through mental processes that are not easy because of their age or illnesses.

Because of the improvement in medical care, nutrition, and sanitary conditions during the last century, we have reached a point where the percentage of elderly in the population has risen steeply, since people live longer than they did in the past. Recently, geriatric science has begun to understand how important human support is in the treatment of these elderly people.

Elderly people, frail-care patients, and chronically ill patients who lie in bed for long periods of time need emotional support, which can be provided partially by aromatherapy. No less important is touch. Regrettably, many elderly people feel that other people are afraid of touching them, as if old age were a contagious disease. Touch is a human need, and the elderly or frail population should not be deprived of it.

It is possible to apply essential oils gently to the patients' bodies. When such a patient is suffering from a disease that does not permit him to be moved so that the oils can be applied to his entire body, we focus on the oil and on performing a local massage – on the face, the neck, or the shoulders. Touch, massage, and caress, mixed with the beneficial, fortifying, and vitality-stimulating fragrance of the oils, induces well-being and joy in elderly or frail-care patients. When people who treat the elderly or frail-care patients include essential oils in their treatments, they report wonderful results.

When treating the elderly and frail-care patients, we must take their low level of vitality into account. Aggressive treatment and treatment with essential oils with a high level of toxicity are not suitable for them.

We must also take into account the fact that these people sometimes take large quantities of medications, and aromatherapy is liable to speed up their elimination from the body. Therefore, if you are not an experienced professional in massage, reflexology, or aromatherapy, you can provide your elderly clients with a great deal of relief and benefit, and make them feel wonderful – without any risk to them – if you place an oil burner containing suitable essential oils in their room. You can use the lists of oils that appeared in the chapters dealing with depression, melancholy, insomnia, anger and confusion, and the instructions for treatment with suitable essential oils presented there.

Another treatment I mentioned at the beginning of the chapter – one that can help raise elderly people's level of vitality and provide a better feeling – is by massaging the face with essential oils (or applying oils to the face). For the massage, we try to use oils with lower levels of toxicity and oils that are suitable for treating infants.

The following oils are suitable: **neroli**, **myrtle**, **lavender**, **niaouli**, **frankincense**, and **chamomile**. Since these oils contain numerous beneficial properties, and are suitable for treating many physical and psychological conditions, they are highly recommended. They are also very gentle oils.

When treating the elderly, it is important to remember to be very gentle. Moreover, when preparing a blend for a facial massage, we must dilute the oils in a larger quantity of carrier oil than usual, in accordance with the client's level of vitality.

In the next section, we will suggest a blend for a facial treatment for (mainly) elderly people, and for treating bedsores.

The rest of the treatments for the elderly, for frail-care patients, or for the seriously ill should be administered by experienced professionals only.

A refreshing facial treatment to make the elderly feel good and cheer them up

Marge, a wonderful woman who spends time treating the elderly population, is an art therapist at a home for the elderly. She works with people who have varying levels of functioning, using movement, music, art, and physiotherapy in movement. She devotes a lot of time and a great deal of soul to her work, and came to me for suggestions for some kind of treatment for the elderly patients in the frail-care unit, some of whom could not participate in the activities offered at the home. She usually spent an hour with these people, during which she read articles from the newspaper and played music to encourage them to join in the community singing, even though they were lying in bed.

She wanted to find another treatment that would give them joy and pleasure.

I recommended that Marge perform a gentle facial massage on both men and women, using a blend of oils that had a beneficial psychological action as well as a refreshing effect on their facial skin.

In the case of this population, it is true to say that any type of touch, not just a caress or a hug, will produce wonderful results from the point of view of how the elderly people feel. Touch, which symbolizes closeness and acceptance, is very important in view of the fact that many frail-care patients feel that they are a burden on society – and sometimes even lose the will to live – both mentally and physically.

I used the following carrier oils in the blend: 10 cc of **apricot kernel oil**, 10 cc of **avocado** oil, 5 cc of **wheatgerm** oil, and 5 cc of **sesame** oil (mainly because of its energetic and warming properties). I added five drops of **evening primrose** oil, which is used for treating irritated, sensitive, and allergic skin, improves skin cell regeneration, and treats damaged, neglected, tired, and old skin.

From among the essential oils, I chose to add three drops of **chamomile**, which is anti-inflammatory, anti-depressant, analgesic, soothing, slightly invigorating, and helps in cases of hypersensitivity; I also added five drops of **lavender** oil, which reinforces the immune system, encourages and improves the mood, soothes, helps promote a feeling of mental balance, and helps treat insomnia; five drops of **frankincense**, which is also a soothing oil, helps treat many respiratory problems with its gentle action, and also promotes a feeling of spiritual openness; and two drops of **marjoram** oil, which helps lower blood pressure, alleviates pains, treats feelings of loneliness and alienation, melancholy and sorrow, gives a feeling of mental warmth, and helps treat insomnia, fatigue, and mental exhaustion.

I used a smaller amount of **marjoram** oil after I found out that there was nobody suffering from critically low blood pressure.

It must be remembered that *the blend for the elderly must be diluted*, as necessary, according to the person's condition.

Marge performed an extremely gentle massage on each of the patients in the frail-care ward. She performed the massage sitting behind or next to the patient's bed, applying the blend gently to the patient's face, very gently massaging the temples, and spreading the blend on the forehead, bridge of the nose and the cheeks – sometimes using slow, soothing movements, and in certain cases using faster and more vigorous movements.

She combined placement of hands in the treatment, and sent the energy of universal love to the patient (Marge has Reiki III qualifications). With certain patients, when possible, she went on to massage their neck, nape and shoulders with gentle movements. The massage took about ten minutes just for the face, and up to 20 minutes for an extremely gentle face, neck, and shoulder massage when the patient's condition permitted.

When she finished the treatments, she was very excited about the success of the massage and the enthusiastic feedback she received from the elderly patients. She said that after the massage, the skin on their faces absolutely glowed. This glow can be attributed to the beneficial action of the carrier and essential oils, but no less, and perhaps even more, to Marge's loving touch, and to the inner glow that she inspired in their hearts.

As a result of the enthusiastic reactions, and the feeling that certain people, who had a tendency toward apathy and indifference, reacted with extraordinary joy to the massage and the touch, Marge decided to make massage a permanent feature, and she gives the frail-care patients a gentle, loving massage once a week, and tries to get other people involved in this worthwhile effort.

Bedsores (mainly in frail-care patients)

Rebecca, who was taking care of her sick father, came to me for help in the treatment of one of the most common problems among patients who hardly get out of bed. Her 83-year-old father had fractured his hip two years before, and his general condition had deteriorated since then. He was now a frail-care patient. Since Rebecca did not work, and her children were grown and no longer needed her ongoing care, she decided to take her father into her home and look after him by herself. (For three hours a day, a frail-care nurse came to wash her father and administer a little bit of basic physiotherapy.) Although her father barely functioned from the physical point of view, his mental functions were relatively good, and she enjoyed being with him.

Despite her devoted care, she discovered that the bedsores from which her father suffered (they had started when he was in the hospital) had not healed. On the contrary, they had worsened. In addition, her father suffered from diabetes, which was treated with pills. The lack of blood supply to the skin exacerbated the bedsores, and a cure was not in the offing.

Bedsores are sores that are first identified as a sensitive, red, and inflamed area on the surface of the skin. Gradually, they become very red, erupt, and become blisters. When the sore becomes a blister, immediate medical intervention is required. Since these sores tend to occur among the population that suffers from a defective blood supply and from a very low skin cell regenerative ability, it takes a long time for them to heal, and sometimes they deteriorate very severely.

Generally, the people who suffer from bedsores are the elderly, diabetics, and people who suffer from blood vessel diseases and lie in bed for extended periods. In people who are comatose, paralyzed, or suffer from diseases that compel them to stay in bed for a long time, the sores appear in the areas that bear the weight of the body – the buttocks, the elbows, the heels, the shoulders, and the hips – or in places where there is constant friction with the pajamas.

Since contact with fluids – sweat and urine – increases the production of bedsores, and sometimes even causes them, it is extremely important to ensure that the patient's hygienic conditions are good, and that his skin is clean and dry. One of the most important ways to prevent bedsores is to change the patient's position very frequently – at least once every two hours – and, when lifting him, not to pull him along the bed, since the friction can aggravate his condition.

A point that is no less important is to help increase the blood flow in the patient's body. If the patient can do various actions by himself, it is important for him to do things such as contracting and relaxing muscles, bending and revolving his elbows, fingers, toes, and ankles, stretching and relaxing his body, and so on.

In these cases, and especially in situations in which the patient cannot move or perform various actions by himself, a massage with essential oils is of utmost importance.

Massage with essential oils helps improve the blood flow in the body and in the area where there are bedsores. In addition, there is a supportive psychological side to the treatment, which gives the patient a feeling of mental warmth and caring and can greatly raise his level of vitality. Since these patients generally have a low level of vitality, the massage with essential oils is performed when the oils are very diluted, and only a quarter of the usual amount of essential oil is used.

The blend I prepared for Rebecca's father contained the following carrier oils: 25 cc of **castor** oil, which is an oil with a low absorptive capacity and is used for treating dry skin, and 5 cc of **wheatgerm** oil, which is rich in vitamin E, is used as an antioxidant, and has a medium absorptive capacity.

The first essential oil I chose to add to the blend was **chamomile** oil (two drops), which is excellent for sensitive, cracked, dry and inflamed skin, and helps in cases of red and irritated skin; it is an antiseptic and a powerful anti-inflammatory, prevents the development of secondary infections, helps heal sores and cuts, purifies and cleanses the blood circulation, and soothes and relieves tension, anxiety and depression. Moreover, **chamomile** is suitable for treating people who are weak or who have a low level of vitality, and contributes to the reinforcement of their immune system.

The second essential oil I added to the blend was **geranium** oil (one drop), which is a disinfectant that is suitable for dry and sensitive skin and very effective for healing sores and blisters on the skin; it soothes inflammations and skin infections, strengthens the skin, cleanses and refreshes it, and is very suitable for mature and old skin.

The third essential oil I added to the blend was **lavender** oil (one drop), which is very important because of its contribution to the reinforcement of the immune system, for the regeneration of the body's tissue cells, for healing sores and infected sores, for soothing irritated skin, and for treating infections and pains generally. It is also important because of its many healing properties and its tendency to treat almost every body system in one way or another – as well as its great effectiveness in balancing various mental states and treating sleep problems, which are common among old patients or among patients who lie in bed for a long time and suffer from a consequent imbalance in their sleeping and waking conditions.

I advised Rebecca to use the blend for massaging the infected areas every day, using slow, light, circular movements. With elderly clients, diabetics or bedridden clients, whose level of vitality is low, it is important to ensure that the massage is not too long. The recommended duration is 10-15 minutes. The massage must be performed with maximum gentleness and with slow, calm movements. A gentle massage means getting the oil to penetrate the skin with massage movements in which very little pressure is exerted, and the massage is more on the surface than in-depth. In fact, when treating clients with a low level of vitality, the massage will fall between a "genuine" massage and simply applying the oil. Frequently, when the client's level of vitality is very low, it is advisable to only apply the blend instead of performing a massage. When in doubt, opt for application of the oil.

Despite his illness, Rebecca's father's vitality was good relative to his condition (thanks to the treatment, the care, and the support he was given). It was therefore possible to treat him with a gentle local massage (that is, not all over his body, but just in the places with bedsores) every day for the first month of treatment. When the level of vitality is lower, the massage or the application should only be done twice or three times a week.

Professional treatment, together with a gentle local massage with essential oils, vastly improved the state of the father's bedsores. There was no occurrence of new bedsores, and the existing ones began to heal, showing a reduction in their inflammation, depth and circumference. In certain areas, the sores healed almost completely, while in others, the extent of their spreading decreased appreciably.

After a month of gentle, daily, 15-minute massages, Rebecca decreased the frequency of the massage to three times a week, mainly in order to maintain the improvement in her father's condition and to prevent the occurrence of new bedsores. She reported that she saw an improvement in her father's vitality, and that the massage with essential oils made him feel better. After the massage, he was in a better mood – sometimes he would even joke and feel cheerful – and he slept better on the days Rebecca had performed the massage. She said that the massage gave him pleasure, and he looked forward eagerly to the next one. At his age and in his condition, where very few things give him pleasure, the importance of the pleasure given by the massage must not be taken lightly.

First Aid

Later on, we will suggest essential oils for several cases that require first aid. We are not talking about heart attacks or traffic accidents, of course, but rather about treating minor things that happen in the home, at work, or outdoors – things that can be relieved or treated by using essential oils, sometimes in conjunction with necessary medical treatment.

Certain oils are good for treating many cases that require first aid, and they should be in every first aid kit at home. Two of the most important essential oils for this purpose are **tea tree** oil and **lavender** oil. These two oils, whose level of toxicity is very low, can be used undiluted (unless otherwise stated on the bottle) for a wide range of bruises, burns, sunburn, cuts, infections, and rashes. **Tea tree** oil is an extraordinary antiseptic, and serves as a powerful and effective disinfectant. **Lavender** oil soothes the skin and promotes tissue regeneration, thereby accelerating the healing of sores and scars.

Marigold oil is also a very effective oil for treating burns, bruises, cuts, and injuries. **Geranium** oil is effective in cases of burns, sunburn, sores and cuts, and disinfects the affected area well.

Superficial cuts and wounds

Because of the powerful antiseptic properties of the oils, they are excellent for treating superficial cuts and wounds. Their disinfectant action is superb, they prevent the development of infections, and they can also help the wound or cut congeal and heal, while either preventing scarring altogether or minimizing it. Remember that if the cut is serious and involves a loss of blood, it must be properly bandaged or it should be stitched up by a physician.

I heard the following stories from my friend Nora, a sculptor and designer who works mainly in wood. One Saturday, a fruitful, idea-filled day for her, she had been sanding a large log for many hours, cutting it with a fret-saw. The work took a long time, but since she was full of creative energy and vitality, she did not stop working until evening. She remembers that she was a bit tired, because working with wood requires physical exertion, and her concentration was not as it had been in the morning. One of the times that she drew the fret-saw across the log, it slipped and cut the first joint of her index finger, causing a large, deep, and bleeding cut that was so deep that the flesh was exposed. Although it is advisable to get medical care for a cut that serious, Nora decided not to stop working. She rinsed off the bleeding wound well, dripped one drop of **lavender** oil and one drop of **tea tree** oil onto it, bandaged her finger carefully, and continued working without paying any attention to the deep cut.

On Monday, the cut was already much better, but it was still deep – almost to the bone – and it was hurting. Nora decided to go and see her physician, who was astounded, and rebuked her for not going to the ER for butterfly stitches (a method of getting the cut to heal using strips of adhesive plaster rather than stitches). "Now it's too late, and you're going to have a serious and ugly scar on your finger…" Nora was sorry that she hadn't gone to the ER immediately, but decided to continue treating the cut with essential oils. Several times a day, she alternately dripped one drop of **tea tree** oil or one drop of **lavender** oil on the cut. To her astonishment, about a week later, the deep wound had healed, and two weeks later, only a scar was visible. She continued the treatment every day, and, within a few weeks, there was only a fine scar on her finger, a thin, almost indiscernible white line around the joint. Today, it is almost impossible to see the scar. (I still think, however, that Nora should have begun the treatment in the ER.)

In many cases, of course, the body has neither the strength nor the ability to heal itself as well as it did in Nora's case, but when treating superficial wounds and cuts, the essential oils are extremely effective.

Tea tree oil is one of the strongest antiseptic oils in existence. Its disinfectant ability is tremendous, it provides a defense against infections, and it helps the wound heal quickly.

Lavender oil is also a wonderful disinfectant, and has regenerative properties that accelerate the renewal of the skin cells, thus helping the wound to knit and heal quickly. **Lavender** oil is also excellent for treating scars, and using it on the cut can greatly reduce the chances of a conspicuous scar remaining.

When treating superficial cuts and wounds, it is also possible to use one drop of **palmarosa** oil, or, *alternatively*, one drop of **geranium** oil, on the wound or cut.

Bruises

After his divorce, Mark, the 42-year-old owner of a clothing store, underwent treatment with Bach flower remedies at the clinic where I worked. One day, I saw him come in with a large, bluish-purple bruise on his forehead. He told me that when he had cleared out the shed at his house (as part of the divorce arrangements), he had become upset and a bit agitated because of all the painful memories that flooded over him, and while he was lost in thought, he carelessly collided with a wooden beam in the shed. Within a short time, a large bruise appeared on his forehead. It hurt him a bit, but he was more concerned about how it looked, since he worked in a store with the public, and it was important for him to look good and presentable.

Bruises are bluish-purple marks, sometimes slightly yellow, that are formed as a result of a blow or a bump that causes damage to the blood vessels in the region. Most bruises heal themselves, without treatment. Sometimes they swell up a bit, and sometimes they hurt – it depends on the person's sensitivity and threshold of pain. Generally, the bruise goes away after a few days, and, if it did not occur in a sensitive place in which it could cause unusual pain, it does not need medical intervention.

People who suffer from diabetes, anemia, or obesity tend to bruise more easily. In diabetics, a bruise, even a small one, can remain on the skin for a long time. In most cases, the bruise is not dangerous (except when it was caused by a very hard blow in a sensitive place, or hurts very significantly for a long time – then it is advisable to check and see if additional damage was caused by the blow), but it can bother the person because of the pain it causes in the region, and what it sometimes looks like.

Treatment with essential oils is very effective in relieving the pain and discoloration of bruises, and can accelerate their healing and disappearance.

I prepared a blend for Mark to apply to the bruise. I warned him not to massage the blend into the bruise, but just to spread it on gently. A bruise must not be massaged, and the sooner it is treated after it occurs, the more effective the treatment with essential oils will be. I used 10 cc of **grapeseed** carrier oil to which I added two drops of **marigold** oil, which is excellent for treating bruises, cuts, and burns, and soothes the area of the injury, two drops of **geranium** oil, and two drops of **parsley** oil, which soothes and helps treat wounds and bruises.

It is important to remember that **parsley** oil *must not be used for treating pregnant women*.

Mark spread the blend gently over the bruise several times a day. He felt fast relief from the pain, and two days later, there was almost no sign of the bruise.

Burns and sunburn

My friend Will owns a yacht and frequently gets sunburned. He is not usually scantily dressed because of his rather sensitive skin, so the sunburn occurs at the back of his neck and sometimes at the sides of his head and below his ears. Will must get into the habit of applying a suitable sunscreen lotion, but sometimes he forgets, and then he pays the price. Once, when he came to visit me, he had a large red patch of sunburn on the back of his neck. "Before you make coffee," he said, "do me a favor and help me get rid of this burn. It bothered me the whole time I was driving to your place, burning and hurting! I need some kind of treatment to soothe the burn."

Sunburn is actually a skin inflammation caused by overexposure to the ultra-violet rays of the sun. In hot climates, sunburn is very common, ranging from mild burns that can be treated at home or with aromatherapy, to serious burns caused by prolonged and significant exposure to the powerful rays of the sun, necessitating medical treatment. Sunburn is seen as hot, red, tender skin, and, in serious cases, blisters on the skin. Sunburn can not only be caused by powerful sunshine, but also by prolonged exposure to medium-strength sunshine. Although there is no significant sensation of burning at the time, some time after the exposure, the sunburn appears. People with fair skin are much more sensitive to the sun, and can suffer from sunburn toward the end of spring and during the summer if they do not make sure to protect themselves against the sun by dressing properly and by using a suitable sunscreen lotion. It must be remembered that recurring sunburn or frequent prolonged exposure to the sun over many years entail a risk of skin cancer. For this reason, the importance of applying sunscreens with suitable protection factors and taking precautions when being exposed to the sun should be recognized.

I recommended that Will use a local treatment that was wonderfully effective.

(It is also suitable for mild burns caused by boiling oil that spatters during cooking, by touching a hot saucepan, and so on).

I rushed over to the first aid closet and took out two wonderful essential oils – pure, undiluted **lavender** and **tea tree** oil – a drop or two (depending on the size of the burn) of which should be spread on the burn immediately, or as soon as possible after the burn occurs. This treatment should be administered every four hours until the condition improves.

I spread a bit of pure **lavender** oil on the large patch of sunburn on Will's neck. After the first application, he did not feel significant relief. Four hours later, I reapplied **lavender** oil to the burn. Before he left, I gave him a bottle of **lavender** oil so that he could continue treating the burn every four hours. The next evening, I got an excited telephone call – the burn had practically disappeared, and no longer hurt. The redness had gone down appreciably, and the circumference of the burn had also greatly decreased. This is not an isolated success in treating sunburn or mild burns with **lavender** and **tea tree** oils.

Essential oils have far-reaching properties in the treatment of infections because of their ability to kill viruses and bacteria. For this reason, they are very important in the treatment of burns, since they prevent infections. In addition, they soothe the skin (especially **lavender** oil), thereby relieving the redness and pain that accompany the burn. Another important property of essential oils in the treatment of burns is their regenerative ability – promoting the production of new skin cells. In this way, the oils bring about a faster rehabilitation of the area of the burn and help prevent marks and scars.

In cases of more serious burns, too, it is possible to treat the affected area – after the burn has "closed" (*under no circumstances before the burn has healed!*) – in order to relieve the pain and promote the fast and effective rehabilitation of the area.

A few months ago, 15-year-old Nicole was burned by boiling water on her upper arm and torso. She underwent medical treatment for the burns, and now, after recovering partially and out of danger, she was still suffering from pain in the area, from intense redness, and from the ugly appearance of the area. The aim of Nicole's treatment was to help relieve the pain as much as possible, at the same time promoting a faster and more effective rehabilitation of her skin.

After consulting with Nicole's physician, who stated that the condition of her burns permitted supplementary treatment by applying essential oils to them, I prepared a blend of oils using four carrier oils:

As a base oil, I chose **almond** oil, of which I used 20 cc. To this, I added 5 cc of **wheatgerm** oil because it is rich in minerals and vitamins (especially vitamin E) that help rehabilitate the skin and soothe the epidermal reactions to the burn; 5 cc of **jojoba** oil, which helps preserve the skin's moisture and improves its elasticity; and 5 drops of **borage** oil, which helps in the regeneration of the skin cells, and helps lower the allergy and sensitivity level of sensitive skin.

To the blend of carrier oils, I added 10 drops of **lavender** oil, whose properties in the treatment of burns and skin rehabilitation have already been described, and five drops of **palmarosa** oil, which is an antiseptic and antiviral oil that promotes the regeneration of the skin cells and rehabilitates the skin.

Nicole's treatment was administered by application only, not by massage, very carefully and gently, so as not to harm the delicate skin and hurt her. We administered the treatment twice a day for three months, but after a fortnight of treatment, it was already possible to see good results in skin rehabilitation. The oils prevented a worsening of the condition due to the development of infections, and gradually contributed to the rehabilitation of the skin and an improvement in its appearance. In addition, they significantly alleviated the pain and soothed the skin. After three months of treatment, the state of her skin had improved appreciably, while a large part of the burn area had been almost entirely rehabilitated.

In order to continue supporting the skin, Nicole was advised to carry on with the treatment with the blend that had been prepared for her, spreading it on the burn area once a day, until she felt that her skin had regained its normal condition and elasticity, and the sensitivity in the burn area had disappeared.

Stings and animal bites

The essential oils, with their powerful disinfectant, antibacterial and antiviral properties, as well as their help in healing wounds and soothing the skin, are very effective when applied to bee stings, mosquito bites, and animal bites.

In these cases, too, the three oils we know from the first aid treatments described previously play a leading role: **lavender** oil, **tea tree** oil, and **geranium** oil.

The following story will illustrate their wonderful effectiveness. During a school trip, 12-year-old Renee was stung by a bee. The area swelled up quickly and hurt intensely, and Renee had a hard time overcoming her pain and her fright. The medic who was accompanying the children on the trip calmed her down, stopped her crying, and extracted the sting (I am not judging his actions, simply relating what he did), but Renee was still in a state of distress.

One of the mothers who was on the trip was familiar with the effectiveness of essential oils in first aid, so she had **lavender** and **tea tree** oils in her backpack. She sat Renee down, applied a bit of pure **lavender** oil to the sting as well as a drop of **lavender** oil behind Renee's ears. The effect of the oil was amazing. Applying oil to the delicate skin behind the ears, through which the oil was absorbed quickly, helped Renee calm down and overcome her fright. The pain in the swollen area gradually decreased, and in a short time, Renee could carry on with the trip, feeling only mild pain.

In any case of a bee sting, annoying mosquito bites, and animal bites, the essential oils help soothe the area and reduce the irritation effectively.

Despite the effective treatment afforded by essential oils, it is very important, in cases of bee stings, to watch out for *signs of an allergic reaction to the sting* – pallor, unusual swelling, excessive sweating, and respiratory difficulties. These signs are likely to lead to anaphylactic shock, a serious allergic reaction of the body to a sting. In such a case, the person must be rushed to the hospital, since he is in danger.

When treating animal bites, the wound must be rinsed well in water, and one of the following oils in its pure form – **geranium**, **lavender**, or **tea tree** – dripped onto it in order to disinfect the bite. It is then important to seek medical treatment in order to make absolutely sure that the animal was not infected with a dangerous disease. This is especially important when the animal in question is not known, or when the bite is serious.

Treating the area of the bite with essential oils disinfects the area well and helps the wound congeal and heal, at the same time preventing scars, or at least conspicuous scars.

Sprains and sprain-like injuries

Anna, a 63-year-old friend of mine, went hiking in the Catskills. Her age notwithstanding, her physical fitness is superb, and she opted for a trip for good hikers. The hike was fantastic, and she enjoyed walking through the enchanted and challenging landscapes en route. The hike, which took place in the fall, took the hikers through muddy terrain, and this required extra caution on their part. Anna slipped once, but got up and continued the hike. The second time she fell, she twisted her ankle severely, and the pain was so intense that the medic bound up her ankle. Anna made her way back to the bus with great difficulty, assisted by two fellow hikers.

A short time later, her ankle began to swell up, change color, and hurt intensely. The next day, Anna's daughter took her to the clinic to have an X-ray. The X-ray revealed that Anna's ankle had not really been sprained. (A sprain occurs when the contact between the tips of the bones is broken, because of a severe blow, and the normal functioning of the joint is jeopardized.) Having said this, many blows do not cause a real sprain in the medical sense, but create symptoms that resemble a sprain – significant swelling, a change of color, an inability to move the area, and intense pain. At the clinic, it transpired that there was no treatment of any kind for Anna's problem, except wearing a tight elastic stocking, and a recommendation to rest with her leg up. However, the pain was very severe and Anna could not walk on her foot. Sometimes the pain was so intense that it radiated to her calf and thigh.

Aromatherapy can treat and help cases of sprains and injuries with symptoms resembling sprains. It is very important to remember that the first thing to do in cases of a serious blow is to bind the place up, try not to move it, and get medical treatment as soon as possible – including an X-ray, in order to ensure that the bone has not been dislocated (and then the physician may return it to its place through manipulation), or that there is no fracture, torn tendon, and so on. After the diagnosis, it is possible to relieve the pains and to expedite the recovery of the injured area with essential oils.

Injuries and sprains must under no circumstances be treated with massage, but rather just by gently applying the blend of oils to the injured area.

Anna asked me to prepare a suitable blend in order to alleviate her severe pain. The most suitable essential oils for treating sprains and sprain-like injuries are **marjoram**, an oil that is used for treating many skeletal and bone problems, **camphor** oil, which is very effective in treating pains in the "movement" system, and **eucalyptus**. It must be remembered that **camphor** oil *must not be used* on asthma sufferers, on pregnant women, or on infants, and, because of its general level of toxicity, it is only suitable for local use, and must not be used in a general body massage.

Anna's treatment, and the treatment of sprains sprain-like injuries in general, can be performed in two stages. In the first stage, it is advisable to use compresses. The treatment with compresses is also suitable for cases in which the spreading of oils is not desirable – such as when the sprain is very serious or the pain is extremely intense. For an acute state of sprain-induced pain, we use a compress of lukewarm (almost cool) water. For the compress, I prepared a neat blend of **camphor**, **eucalyptus**, and **marjoram** oils.

The blend, in a small bottle, contained 12 drops of **marjoram** oil, six drops of **camphor** oil, and eight drops of **eucalyptus** oil, and this amount was sufficient for many compresses. Two to three drops of the pure oil blend are added to one quart of lukewarm-cool water; cotton or clean cotton fabric is soaked in the water, wrung out slightly, and placed on the affected area for 15 minutes. (In the case of children, the quantities of oil are less.)

I advised Anna to use the compress three times a day for the first two days. She placed the compress and felt a decrease in swelling and pain. When the pain diminished a bit, and it was possible to touch her ankle, I began treatment by spreading the oil. To that end, I prepared a blend of carrier and essential oils. I used 25 cc of **grapeseed** carrier oil and 5 cc of **olive** carrier oil, which is very effective in the treatment of sprains. I added six drops of **marjoram** oil, three drops of **camphor** oil, and four drops of **eucalyptus** oil. Anna's daughter volunteered to apply the blend gently and carefully to Anna's ankle twice a day, until the pains receded. The application significantly relieved the pains in Anna's ankle. The swelling went down, and within a week, Anna was able to walk on her foot without feeling severe pain. I suggested that she not tire her leg, and that she continue applying oil to her ankle once or twice a day for the next week, so as to help the area heal completely.

Blisters

Bill, a 19-year-old cadet at a prestigious military academy, came for treatment with aromatherapy as a result of a very common problem among the military – blisters. Blisters can form as an allergic reaction of injured skin, or as a result of a burn or friction. Blisters look like an accumulation of fluids under the skin. The fluid in the blister is absorbed into the skin, while below the blister new layers of skin are formed, and the outer layer of skin peels off.

Bill had a number of blisters on various parts of his feet following a long march. The blisters burned and stung, and interfered with his regular walking. When he came home on furlough, I advised him to drip one or two drops of one of the following pure essential oils on the blisters: **geranium**, **lavender**, or **tea tree**, or to spread the oil on them gently using a cotton-tipped swab.

One of the blisters had been chafed repeatedly because of the march. It had torn, exposing the skin beneath it, and this caused Bill intense pain and burning. When treating blisters, it is important to remember that the top layer of skin must not be peeled off, since that only makes the area susceptible to additional infection. In this case, I was afraid that the open blister had become infected, and for that reason, it was necessary to drip **tea tree** oil on it in order to disinfect it effectively. After doing so, I covered the blister with a sterile pad so as to prevent further chafing and the worsening of the condition. (In principle, it is not advisable to cover a blister that has burst, and it is preferable to disinfect it and air the foot, but if there is a fear that it will become infected or be subjected to additional chafing, it should be covered carefully with a sterile pad.)

I asked Bill to see that he aired his foot properly while he was on furlough, and to drip **tea tree** oil on the blisters twice a day.

To his great joy, the burning sensation in the blisters ceased to a large extent, and two days later, they were much better. The blister that had burst did not become infected, thanks to proper treatment, and healed quickly.

People in the military or people going on long treks should take a bottle of **tea tree** oil with them. It is extremely effective in disinfecting blisters and soothing the burning (as are **lavender** and **geranium** oils), for ensuring rapid healing of the skin in cases of burst blisters, and for preventing burst blisters from becoming infected. Moreover, the oil helps in effectively treating and disinfecting many cuts, chafed areas, or sores that have become infected.